The Daydream Trap

Break Free from Maladaptive Daydreaming with Acceptance and Commitment Therapy (ACT) and Somatic Tools to Reclaim Your Present Life

Essie Lindsey Haley

First Edition: 2025

ISBN: 978-1-7643782-3-9

Table of Contents

Introduction: A Prisoner of Your Own Mind?

You're supposed to be working on that report. The one that's been sitting on your desk for three days. But instead, you're somewhere else entirely.

You're the lead singer of a band, taking the stage in front of thousands. The lights hit your face. The crowd roars. Your best friend—the one you lost touch with years ago—is in the front row, tears streaming down their face, finally seeing who you really are. Or maybe you're not a rock star at all. Maybe you're the hero who just saved the city, or the brilliant scientist making a groundbreaking discovery, or the person who finally said exactly the right thing to that family member who never understood you.

Two hours pass. Sometimes four. Sometimes more.

When you finally snap back, the report is still blank. Your coffee is cold. And that feeling hits—the one that's become all too familiar. Shame. Frustration. The sickening realization that you just lost another chunk of your life to something you can't quite explain to anyone else.

"I was just daydreaming," doesn't capture it. Because this isn't the gentle mind-wandering that happens when you're stuck in traffic or waiting for water to boil. This is different. This is *consuming*. This feels more real than real life. And stopping it feels about as easy as holding your breath for an hour.

If you're reading this, you probably know exactly what I'm talking about.

1

What This Book Is Really About

Let's get something straight right now. This isn't a book about killing your imagination. Your ability to create these rich, detailed inner worlds? That's not the problem. The problem is that these worlds have become more appealing, more satisfying, and frankly more *manageable* than the actual life you're living.

You're not lazy. You're not weak. You don't lack discipline or willpower.

What you have is something called **Maladaptive Daydreaming**, and it's exactly what it sounds like—daydreaming that's gotten so intense, so time-consuming, and so difficult to control that it's interfering with your real life. The term was coined by researcher Eli Somer in 2002 when he noticed a pattern in some of his patients: they were spending hours each day in elaborate fantasy worlds, often triggered by specific things like music or repetitive movements, and they felt genuinely distressed about their inability to stop (Somer, 2002).

Here's what makes it so confusing: for most of your life, you've probably been told that having a vivid imagination is a *good* thing. Creative. Special. A sign of intelligence. And in many ways, that's true. But somewhere along the line, this gift turned into something else. The fantasies that used to be fun started eating up hours of your day. The daydreams that helped you cope with a boring commute now keep you from doing basic tasks. The inner world that used to feel like a pleasant escape now feels like a trap you can't get out of.

And here's the part that probably makes you feel most alone: when you try to explain this to people, they don't get it. "Just stop daydreaming," they say, as if you hadn't thought of that. "Just focus." "Just be present." As if it were that simple. As if you could just flip a switch and turn off this part of your brain that's been running at full speed for years, maybe decades.

(If one more person tells you to "just be more mindful," you might scream. I get it.)

The Shame No One Talks About

You've probably kept this pretty quiet. Maybe you've mentioned it to one or two people, testing the waters, but their blank stares or confused responses shut you down fast. So you learned to hide it. You got good at looking like you're paying attention in meetings while you're actually finishing Chapter 47 of your ongoing mental saga. You mastered the art of the understanding nod while your mind is entirely somewhere else.

But keeping it secret makes it worse, doesn't it? Because now you're carrying around this huge part of your life that no one knows about. You're mourning the loss of entire afternoons to fantasies while simultaneously feeling like you can't tell anyone because they'll think you're strange. Or worse—they'll think you're just making excuses for being unproductive.

The shame builds. You start wondering if there's something fundamentally broken about you. You watch other people seemingly handle their lives with ease—showing up, doing the work, being present—and you can't figure out why you can't do the same. You buy planners and productivity apps. You try meditation. You promise yourself that tomorrow will be different, that you'll finally get control of this thing.

And then tomorrow comes. The music starts. Your mind drifts. And there you go again.

Here's what you need to hear: **This isn't a character flaw. This is a coping mechanism that's outlived its usefulness.**

At some point, probably years ago, your mind figured out that these fantasies provided something your real life wasn't giving you. Maybe it was escape from boredom, anxiety, or loneliness.

3

Maybe it was a way to feel successful when real life kept knocking you down. Maybe it was the only place where you could feel truly understood, truly powerful, truly *yourself*. Your brain latched onto this strategy because it *worked*. The fantasies gave you relief, excitement, connection—all the things humans desperately need.

The problem is that your brain got too good at it. What started as an occasional escape became the main event. The fantasy world started providing such reliable hits of good feelings that real life couldn't compete. And now you're stuck in what researchers call a "behavioral addiction"—your brain has learned that the fastest, most reliable way to feel good is to check out and drift into your inner world (Somer, Lehrfeld, Bigelsen, & Jopp, 2016).

But here's the thing that might surprise you: **You don't have to destroy your imagination to get your life back.**

Why "Just Stop" Doesn't Work

Before we go any further, let's deal with the advice that everyone (including you) has probably tried: just stopping.

"Stop daydreaming." "Stay focused." "Be present." Sounds reasonable, right? Except it doesn't work. And if you've been beating yourself up because you can't seem to "just stop," you can let that go right now. Because trying to white-knuckle your way out of maladaptive daydreaming is like trying to cure anxiety by telling yourself to "just calm down." It ignores how the brain actually works.

Here's why: your daydreams aren't random mental static. They're serving a function. They're meeting needs. When you try to simply stop without addressing those needs or building alternatives, your brain panics. It's like taking away someone's pain medication without giving them anything else for the pain.

4

Of course they're going to crave it. Of course they're going to go back to it.

Think about it this way. You're stressed at work, and you've trained your brain that the fastest way to feel better is to slip into a fantasy where you're successful and admired. Now imagine trying to "just stop" doing that. Your brain is like, "Wait, but we're stressed. We need relief. The fantasy is right there. Why aren't we using it?" The urge becomes overwhelming. And when you give in (which you will, because you're human), you feel like you've failed. Which makes you feel worse. Which makes you want to escape into fantasy even more.

See the loop?

Plus—and this is important—**trying to suppress thoughts makes them stronger**. There's famous research by Daniel Wegner where he told people not to think about white bears, and guess what happened? They couldn't stop thinking about white bears (Wegner, Schneider, Carter, & White, 1987). The harder they tried not to think about it, the more the white bears dominated their thoughts. Your daydreams work the same way. The harder you fight them, the more powerful they become.

So if willpower doesn't work, what does?

The Anchor & Pivot Model: A Different Approach

This book is built on a simple but powerful idea: **You can't just stop something without starting something else.**

You need two skills, not one. You need a way to *interrupt* the drift when it happens (that's the **Anchor**), and you need a reason to *want* to stay in real life (that's the **Pivot**). Most approaches to this problem focus on one or the other. They either teach you to "be present" without giving you any reason why you'd want to be, or they tell you to "build a better life" without giving you the skills to stay focused long enough to build anything.

You need both.

Let me break it down.

The Anchor is your "stop" button—but it's not about stopping thoughts. It's about learning to notice when you're drifting and gently pulling your attention back to your physical body and the present moment. This uses somatic (body-based) tools that are simple, fast, and surprisingly effective. We're talking 30-second interventions. Noticing the feeling of your feet on the floor. Taking three deep breaths. Naming five things you can see in the room. These techniques work because they shift your attention from your mind (where the fantasy lives) to your body (which exists only in the here and now). Your body is the anchor that keeps you tethered to reality.

The Pivot is your "go" button. This is where we use principles from Acceptance and Commitment Therapy (ACT), which is all about building a life based on your values—the things that really matter to you. Here's the truth: if your real life feels empty, boring, or meaningless, no amount of "anchoring" will help. You'll just keep drifting back because the fantasy is more appealing. The Pivot teaches you how to identify what your daydreams are really giving you (connection? competence? recognition?) and then build those things into your actual life in small, doable ways.

The Anchor gets you *out* of the fantasy. The Pivot gives you somewhere *to go*.

And here's what makes this different from everything else you've tried: **we're not trying to kill your creativity. We're trying to redirect it.**

That incredibly powerful imagination of yours? It's not going anywhere. But instead of letting it use you—stealing your time, your focus, your ability to build the life you actually want— you're going to learn how to use it. On purpose. For things that matter. We'll even set aside time for you to daydream intentionally, because fighting your nature is exhausting and doesn't work anyway.

But you'll be in charge. Not your fantasies.

What to Expect from This Book

Here's how this is going to work. We're going to start by understanding what you're dealing with—what maladaptive daydreaming actually is, why the drift is so powerful, and why your usual strategies haven't worked. That's Part 1. We need to understand the problem before we can fix it.

Then we're moving into the practical stuff: the Anchor & Pivot Toolkit. This is a six-step plan that will teach you how to catch the drift early, pull yourself back to the present moment, unhook from the stories your mind tells you, identify what you really need, and start building a real life that's actually compelling. That's Part 2, and it's where the real work happens.

Finally, we'll talk about what life looks like on the other side— not a life without daydreams, but a life where you're in control. Where you can use your imagination when you want to, for things that matter, instead of losing hours to it against your will. That's Part 3.

Each chapter includes exercises and worksheets. (Yeah, I know, homework. But trust me on this—reading about these tools won't change anything. You have to practice them.) The exercises are short and practical. No complicated meditation routines or hour-long journaling sessions. Just simple, concrete actions you can take today.

One more thing: this process isn't going to be perfect. You're going to drift. You're going to lose entire afternoons to fantasy even after you've learned these tools. That's normal. That's part of being human. We're not shooting for perfection. We're shooting for progress. We're shooting for a life where the fantasy doesn't run the show anymore.

So if you're ready—if you're tired of living in your head and you want to build something real—let's get started.

Your life is waiting for you. And I promise, it can be just as interesting as the one you've been imagining.

Chapter 1: Recognizing Maladaptive Daydreaming

Sarah sits at her desk, staring at the spreadsheet that's been open on her screen for 45 minutes. She hasn't entered a single number. Instead, she's been running through the same scene in her mind for what feels like the hundredth time: the conversation where she finally tells off her boss, except in this version, she's articulate and confident, and everyone in the office applauds as she walks out. She knows this fantasy by heart now. Every line of dialogue. Every facial expression. Every dramatic pause.

Her phone buzzes. It's her reminder to pick up her daughter from soccer practice. She looks at the clock. How did an hour pass? She was only going to "think for a minute."

This happens three or four times a day. Sometimes more.

Is this normal daydreaming? Or is it something else?

Here's the short answer: **It's something else.**

But before you panic or feel even more broken than you already do, let's talk about what makes maladaptive daydreaming different from the regular mental wandering that everyone experiences. Because there *is* a difference, and understanding it is the first step to doing something about it.

Daydreaming and Maladaptive Daydreaming

Everyone daydreams. Your coworker spaces out during the boring parts of meetings. Your friend gets lost in thought on long drives. Your partner stares out the window sometimes, clearly somewhere else mentally. This is totally normal. The human mind wanders. Studies suggest that people spend about 47% of their waking hours thinking about something other than what they're currently doing (Killingsworth & Gilbert, 2010). Almost half! So if your mind drifts occasionally, you're in good company.

But what you're experiencing isn't occasional. It's not a brief mental vacation. It's an *immersive, compulsive, time-consuming alternative reality* that you can't easily control.

Here's how you know the difference. Regular daydreaming:

- Happens spontaneously and ends naturally
- Usually lasts a few seconds to a few minutes
- Doesn't interfere with your ability to function
- Can be redirected without much effort
- Doesn't cause significant distress

Maladaptive daydreaming:

- Happens in response to specific triggers (we'll get to those in a minute)
- Can last for hours at a time
- Actively interferes with work, relationships, and daily responsibilities
- Feels nearly impossible to stop once it starts
- Causes real distress because you can't seem to control it

The word *maladaptive* is key here. It means that something that could be helpful in small doses has become harmful because it's excessive or out of control. Your daydreaming has crossed the line from "creative mental break" to "serious problem that's eating up your life."

And yeah, that's a hard thing to admit. But you're here, reading this book, which means you're already brave enough to face it.

The Five Key Signs of Maladaptive Daydreaming

Eli Somer's research identified several characteristics that separate maladaptive daydreaming from normal fantasy. Not everyone has all of these, but if you're recognizing three or more, you're probably dealing with MD (Somer, 2002; Somer et al., 2016).

1. Your Daydreams Are Vivid and Narrative-Driven

This isn't vague, fuzzy thinking. These are *movies* in your head. Detailed, complex, ongoing storylines with characters, dialogue, plot twists, and emotional depth. You're not just randomly imagining things. You're living in a fully developed alternative world that has continuity from one session to the next.

Marcus, a 32-year-old software developer, described his daydreams this way: "I have an entire universe in my head. There are about twenty main characters, and I know their backstories, their relationships, their motivations. The 'plot' has been going for over ten years now. Sometimes I pick up right where I left off, like turning on a TV show. Other times I rewind and replay scenes I particularly liked, changing small details to see how it affects the outcome."

That level of detail? That's MD.

Your daydreams probably have recurring themes, too. Maybe you're always the hero. Maybe you're always in a romantic relationship with someone who truly understands you. Maybe you're always successful, admired, powerful. These aren't random fantasies—they're carefully constructed worlds where you get to be the person you wish you were or have the experiences you wish you were having.

2. You Have Repetitive Triggers

Here's where it gets really specific. Most people with MD can identify exact triggers that pull them into the daydream state. Common ones include:

- **Music**: Certain songs or genres send you straight into fantasy mode. Sometimes you deliberately put on that music because you *want* to drift. Other times you hear it accidentally and boom—you're gone.
- **Repetitive movement**: Pacing back and forth. Rocking. Swinging your leg. Twirling your hair. These physical actions often accompany the daydreams and can actually trigger them. Some people can't daydream *without* moving.
- **Being alone**: The moment you're by yourself, the daydreams kick in. It's almost automatic. You might even avoid social situations because you're craving alone time to get back to your fantasy.
- **Specific locations**: Your bed, the shower, a particular chair, a long commute. These places become associated with daydreaming, and your brain goes into autopilot when you're there.
- **Boredom or understimulation**: Any dull task—folding laundry, sitting in traffic, waiting in line—becomes a doorway to your fantasy world.
- **Stress or emotional pain**: When real life gets hard, the fantasy is always there as an escape hatch.

The trigger-response pattern is crucial. Regular daydreaming happens randomly. Maladaptive daydreaming happens *on cue*, almost like a reflex. You put on your headphones and start walking, and before you've consciously decided to daydream, you're already deep in the story.

3. You Feel Distressed About the Time You're Losing

This is what separates MD from just being a creative person who likes to imagine things. **You're upset about it.** You don't want to be spending this much time in fantasy. You're aware that it's a problem. You've tried to stop, or at least cut back, and you can't.

You might feel:

- **Guilt** about "wasting" hours when you could be working, socializing, or accomplishing something
- **Shame** about not being able to control your own mind
- **Frustration** because you keep promising yourself you'll stop, but you don't
- **Fear** that this is going to ruin your career, your relationships, or your future
- **Grief** over lost time and missed opportunities

This distress is what makes it *maladaptive*. If you were happily daydreaming for hours and it wasn't causing any problems in your life, this would just be an interesting personality quirk. But you're not happy about it. You recognize that something is wrong. You want things to be different.

And that awareness, painful as it is, is actually a good sign. It means you haven't completely checked out. Part of you still cares about building a real life.

4. It's Interfering with Your Real Life

Let's be blunt. Your daydreaming is costing you something. Maybe a lot of somethings.

At work, you're underperforming. Projects take twice as long as they should because you keep spacing out. You've missed deadlines. You sit through meetings without absorbing a word. Your boss has noticed that you seem "distracted" or "not fully engaged," and you don't know how to explain that you're not distracted—you're *somewhere else entirely*.

In relationships, you're only half-present. Your partner or friends think you're a good listener, but really you're just nodding while continuing the mental narrative in your head. You cancel plans because you'd rather stay home and daydream. You've been told you're "hard to reach" or "in your own world," and both of those things are uncomfortably accurate.

Some people with MD report that their fantasy world is so satisfying that real relationships feel disappointing by comparison. Real people are unpredictable, complicated, and sometimes boring. The people in your head are exactly who you need them to be, every single time.

Your responsibilities pile up. The laundry doesn't get done. The dishes sit in the sink. You meant to pay that bill three days ago, but you've been busy (busy in your head, at least). Your life starts to look chaotic, not because you can't manage basic tasks, but because the tasks keep getting pushed aside for "just five more minutes" in the fantasy—which turns into five hours.

This is serious. When your daydreaming is actively preventing you from functioning in the real world, it's crossed the line from harmless to harmful.

5. It Feels Compulsive and Difficult to Control

Here's maybe the most frustrating part: **You can't seem to stop, even when you want to.**

You tell yourself you're going to focus today. You really need to finish that assignment. You set a timer, you put away your headphones, you sit down with good intentions. And somehow, 20 minutes later, you realize you've been staring at the same paragraph while mentally replaying your favorite fantasy scene. You didn't consciously choose to drift. It just happened.

Or you *do* manage to pull yourself out, but the urge to go back is so strong that you can't concentrate on anything else. It's like trying to diet while someone holds a chocolate cake in front of your face. The pull is constant, exhausting, overwhelming.

Some people describe it as an addiction, and research is starting to back that up. Studies have found similarities between MD and behavioral addictions like gambling or compulsive internet use (Somer, Soffer-Dudek, & Ross, 2017). The same reward circuits in your brain light up. The same cravings, the same inability to stop despite negative consequences, the same feeling of needing it to cope with stress.

This isn't about being weak-willed. Your brain has learned that daydreaming provides fast, reliable relief from discomfort and a quick hit of good feelings. Once that pattern is established, it's genuinely hard to break. Not impossible—we're going to work on that—but hard enough that you can't just "decide" to stop and have it stick.

But Here's the Other Side: You're Also Creative, Empathetic, and Searching for Meaning

Before we go any further, I need you to understand something that often gets lost when people talk about maladaptive daydreaming. **Your ability to create these elaborate inner worlds is actually a sign of some pretty remarkable strengths.**

Yes, it's causing problems right now. Yes, we need to address that. But the same mental capacities that enable MD are the same ones that make you:

Highly creative: The level of detail and complexity in your daydreams requires serious imaginative horsepower. You're essentially writing novels in your head, complete with character development, plot arcs, and emotional depth. That's not nothing. That's a genuine creative gift.

Deeply empathetic: Many people with MD create rich emotional landscapes in their fantasies. You can imagine exactly how your characters feel, what they need, why they act the way they do. You can step into multiple perspectives. This capacity for empathy is valuable, even if right now it's pointed inward rather than outward.

Hungry for meaning: Your daydreams aren't random. They're about something. Usually they're about being competent, connected, understood, successful—all the core human needs that drive us to build lives worth living. The fact that you're seeking these things, even in fantasy form, means you *want* a meaningful existence. You haven't given up on that. You've just been trying to find it in the wrong place.

Researchers have found that people with MD often score high on measures of creativity and absorption (the ability to become deeply immersed in experiences) (Bigelsen, Lehrfeld, Jopp, & Somer, 2016). These are traits associated with artists, writers, and innovators. In the right context, with the right tools, your imaginative capacity could be channeled into something genuinely productive and fulfilling.

So here's what I want you to hear: **We're not trying to kill the part of you that imagines. We're trying to redirect it.**

You don't need to become some boring, uncreative robot who only thinks about spreadsheets. You need to learn how to use your imagination intentionally, for things that matter, instead of letting it run wild and consume your life. There's a big difference between "spending two hours building a fantasy world in your head while your real responsibilities crumble" and "spending 30 minutes deliberately planning a creative project, then taking action on it."

One is MD. The other is just being a creative person.

We're going to get you from the first to the second.

Worksheet: Your Daydreaming Profile

Alright, time to get specific about your own patterns. This isn't about judging yourself. It's about gathering data. You can't change what you don't understand, so we're going to map out exactly what your MD looks like.

Grab a notebook or open a document on your computer. Answer these questions as honestly as you can. No one else needs to see this. This is just for you.

Part 1: Your Triggers

What specific things tend to trigger your daydreaming? Check all that apply and add any others:

- Specific songs or music genres (list them)
- Being alone
- Repetitive movements (which ones?)
- Specific locations (where?)
- Boredom or dull tasks
- Stress or anxiety
- Feeling lonely or misunderstood
- Right before bed or first thing in the morning
- Other: _____

Which trigger is the *strongest*—the one that almost always pulls you into fantasy?

Part 2: Your Main Plots

What are the recurring themes in your daydreams? Don't overthink this. Just describe what tends to happen:

- Are you usually the main character?
- What kind of person are you in the daydreams? (heroic, romantic, successful, powerful, understood, etc.)
- Are there recurring "scenes" or storylines you return to over and over?
- Do you have specific characters who appear regularly?
- What feelings do these daydreams give you? (excitement, peace, satisfaction, connection, etc.)

Part 3: The Time Cost

Be honest. How much time are you actually losing to this?

- How many hours per day do you estimate you spend daydreaming?
- What activities or responsibilities are you neglecting because of it?
- When was the last time you lost track of several hours to daydreaming?
- What's the longest single "session" you can remember?

Part 4: The Impact

What is this costing you? Again, be honest:

- How is it affecting your work or school performance?
- How is it affecting your relationships?
- How is it affecting your physical health (sleep, exercise, eating)?
- How is it affecting your mental health (stress, guilt, shame)?
- What opportunities have you missed because you were daydreaming instead of taking action?

Part 5: What You've Already Tried

What strategies have you attempted to control this? (e.g., avoiding triggers, setting timers, meditation, therapy, etc.)

What worked, even a little bit?

What didn't work at all?

Take your time with this. The clearer you can be about your own patterns, the easier it will be to apply the tools we're going to learn. There's no judgment here. You're just collecting information about how your brain works so you can start working *with* it instead of fighting against it.

What You've Learned So Far

Maladaptive daydreaming isn't just creativity or a vivid imagination. It's an intense, time-consuming pattern that interferes with real life and causes genuine distress. You're not imagining things (pun intended)—this is a real phenomenon with specific characteristics.

You now know the five key signs: vivid narrative daydreams, repetitive triggers, distress about lost time, interference with daily functioning, and difficulty controlling the urge. If you recognized yourself in most or all of these, you're dealing with MD. And that means you're not alone in this.

You've also started mapping your own patterns—your triggers, your plots, the time you're losing, and the impact it's having. This information is going to be crucial as we move forward. Because you can't change patterns you don't understand.

But here's the most important thing you learned in this chapter: **Your imagination isn't the enemy. The lack of control is.** You have genuine creative strengths that are currently being misused. We're going to fix that.

In the next chapter, we'll talk about *why* the drift is so powerful—what your daydreams are really doing for you, and why trying to "just stop" keeps failing. Understanding the function of your MD is the key to changing it.

Chapter 2: Why Is the "Drift" So Powerful?

Let's start with a question you've probably asked yourself a thousand times: *Why can't I just stop?*

You're not stupid. You know the daydreaming is a problem. You can see the consequences piling up—the missed deadlines, the strained relationships, the opportunities slipping away. You've tried to quit. Multiple times. You've deleted the playlists that trigger you, you've avoided being alone, you've thrown yourself into work with renewed determination. And yet, within days (sometimes hours), you're back in the fantasy.

What gives?

Here's the answer that might surprise you: **Your daydreams are working perfectly.** They're doing exactly what your brain designed them to do. The problem isn't that they don't work. The problem is that they work *too well*.

To understand what I mean, we need to talk about the *function* of behavior. This is a concept from behavioral psychology, and it's simple but powerful: every behavior serves a purpose, even destructive ones. People don't do things randomly. They do things because those things provide some kind of payoff—usually either escaping something unpleasant or gaining something desirable (Cooper, Heron, & Heward, 2020).

Your maladaptive daydreaming? It's serving both functions simultaneously. It's helping you escape discomfort *and* giving you access to feelings of fulfillment that your real life isn't providing. That's a hell of a one-two punch. No wonder it's so hard to give up.

Let's break down exactly what your daydreams are doing for you—and why that makes them so maddeningly difficult to stop.

Function #1: Escape from Discomfort

Think about when you're most likely to drift into fantasy. I'm willing to bet it's not when you're genuinely excited, engaged, and energized by what's happening in real life. It's when you're:

Bored. Sitting through a tedious meeting. Doing repetitive tasks. Waiting for something to happen. Stuck in traffic. Your brain is understimulated, desperate for something interesting, and the fantasy world is right there, always ready with excitement and drama.

Anxious. Worrying about an upcoming conversation, a looming deadline, a social situation you're dreading. The fantasy offers immediate relief. In your daydream, you're confident, articulate, in control. The real-world anxiety fades into the background, at least temporarily.

Lonely. Maybe you're physically alone, or maybe you're surrounded by people who don't really *get* you. Either way, you feel disconnected and isolated. And in the fantasy? You're deeply understood. You have meaningful connections. Someone sees the real you and loves what they see.

Inadequate. You just failed at something, or you're facing a task you don't think you can handle, or you're comparing yourself to others and coming up short. The fantasy lets you be competent, successful, admired. You get to be the version of yourself you wish you were.

Overwhelmed. Life feels like too much. Too many demands, too many responsibilities, too many decisions. The fantasy is simple and controllable. You're in charge of the plot. Nothing happens that you don't want to happen.

22

See the pattern? Every single one of these is an *uncomfortable emotional state*. And your brain, which is fundamentally in the business of avoiding discomfort, has learned that daydreaming is the fastest route to relief.

This is important to understand: **You're not escaping reality for no reason. You're escaping because reality feels bad.**

And here's the thing—this strategy actually makes sense. Humans have always used imagination to cope with difficult situations. Prisoners of war have survived torture by retreating into elaborate mental worlds. People going through medical procedures manage pain by visualizing themselves somewhere else. Kids in chaotic homes create fantasy friends for comfort. Mental escape is a legitimate survival tool.

The problem is that your brain has generalized this tool to *all* discomfort, not just genuine threats. Bored in a meeting? Fantasy. Nervous about a date? Fantasy. Lonely on a Friday night? Fantasy. The neural pathway from "uncomfortable feeling" to "initiate daydream" has been so well-worn that it's become automatic. You don't even consciously decide to drift anymore. You just... do.

Psychologists call this *negative reinforcement*, which is a terrible name because it sounds like it's about punishment, but actually it means that a behavior is strengthened by the removal of something unpleasant (Skinner, 1953). Every time you escape discomfort by daydreaming, the behavior gets reinforced. Your brain learns: *Feeling bad? Daydream. Problem solved. Do it again next time.*

And you do. Over and over and over. Until the escape hatch becomes the main exit you use for everything.

Function #2: The Search for Fulfillment

But escape is only half the story. If daydreaming just helped you avoid pain, you might not be so hooked. The real power of MD comes from what it gives you: a sense of fulfillment.

Let's get specific about what "fulfillment" means. According to Self-Determination Theory, a well-researched framework in psychology, humans have three basic psychological needs (Ryan & Deci, 2000):

Competence: The need to feel effective, capable, and skilled at what you do **Connection**: The need for meaningful relationships and a sense of belonging **Autonomy**: The need for control over your own life and choices

When these needs are met in real life, people thrive. When they're not met, people struggle—and they often turn to substitutes that provide the *feeling* of fulfillment without the actual thing.

Like, say, elaborate fantasy worlds.

Now think about the content of your daydreams. What role do you typically play?

The hero who saves the day? That's competence. You're skilled, effective, important. People depend on you, and you come through.

The person in a perfect romantic relationship? That's connection. You're seen, understood, loved unconditionally.

The successful artist/athlete/businessperson who gets recognition? That's both competence (you're good at what you do) and connection (people admire and appreciate you).

24

The person who makes their own decisions and isn't controlled by anyone? That's autonomy. You're in charge. You call the shots.

Your daydreams aren't random wish fulfillment. They're very specifically designed to meet the psychological needs that your real life isn't meeting. **Your fantasies are showing you what you're hungry for.**

And here's why this matters: these needs are legitimate. There's nothing wrong with wanting to feel competent, connected, and autonomous. In fact, those desires are *healthy*. They're what drive people to learn skills, build relationships, and create meaningful lives. The problem isn't the needs themselves. The problem is that you're trying to satisfy them in a way that doesn't actually work.

It's like being hungry and smelling cookies baking. The smell gives you a little hit of satisfaction, but it doesn't fill your stomach. Your fantasy world is the smell of cookies. It activates the same brain regions associated with real fulfillment, but it doesn't provide the actual nutrition your psyche needs.

Researchers have found that people with MD often have a particular psychological profile: they're highly imaginative, have a strong need for emotional stimulation, and often feel that real life doesn't meet their needs for excitement or meaning (Somer et al., 2016). That last part is crucial. You're not daydreaming just because you *can*. You're daydreaming because reality feels insufficient.

So your brain says, "Okay, we need fulfillment. We're not getting it in real life. But we can get a simulacrum of it in the fantasy world. Let's go there instead."

And it works. Sort of. For a little while. Until the fantasy ends and you're back in real life, which still isn't giving you what you need. So you go back to the fantasy. Again and again.

The Addictive Loop: Why One Hit Is Never Enough

Now here's where things get really tricky. You might have noticed that your daydreaming operates on a familiar cycle:

The Trigger: Something happens—you put on music, you're alone, you're stressed.

The Urge: You feel a strong pull toward the fantasy. It's almost physical, like hunger or thirst.

The Behavior: You give in and drift into the daydream. For a while, it feels great. You get relief from discomfort plus a hit of fulfillment. This is the *reward*.

The Crash: Eventually, you snap back to reality. The work still isn't done. The problem you were avoiding is still there. And now you've also got guilt and shame about the time you just lost. You feel *worse* than before.

The New Trigger: That worse feeling (guilt, anxiety, self-loathing) becomes a new trigger. And what's your brain's favorite strategy for escaping uncomfortable feelings? More daydreaming.

This is what addiction specialists call a *reinforcement cycle*, and it's how behavioral addictions maintain themselves (Griffiths, 2005). The behavior provides immediate relief and pleasure, which reinforces doing it again. But it also creates new problems (lost time, increased stress, shame), which *also* trigger more of the behavior. You're caught in a loop where the solution to the problem caused by daydreaming is... more daydreaming.

Here's what makes it even more insidious: **the fantasy is designed to be more rewarding than real life.**

In your daydreams, everything goes exactly how you want it to. You always say the perfect thing. People always respond the way you hope they will. You never fail, never embarrass yourself, never have to deal with uncertainty or rejection. The reward is *instant* and *reliable*.

Compare that to real life. You ask someone out—maybe they say yes, maybe they don't. You try to learn a new skill—it takes weeks or months before you feel competent. You reach out to a friend—they might be busy or distracted or just not that interested. Real life is slow, unpredictable, and full of failure. The rewards are uncertain and delayed.

Your brain, which is fundamentally lazy and designed to seek the path of least resistance, looks at these two options and thinks, "Yeah, fantasy please."

Neuroscientist Judson Brewer explains that our brains are constantly running a reward-based learning system: we do something, we get a result, and our brains encode whether that result was good or bad (Brewer, 2017). The actions that produce good results get prioritized. The actions that produce bad results get avoided. Daydreaming produces fast, reliable, powerful good feelings. Engaging with real life produces slow, uncertain, mixed results. Is it any wonder your brain keeps choosing the fantasy?

This is why willpower doesn't work. You're not fighting against a bad habit. You're fighting against your brain's fundamental programming to seek reward and avoid discomfort. And as long as the fantasy provides better rewards than real life, your brain is going to keep choosing it.

Why Your Brain Won't Let You "Just Stop"

Let's return to that original question: why can't you just stop?

Because **stopping would mean sitting with the discomfort the daydreams are helping you avoid, while also giving up the sense of fulfillment the daydreams are providing, without having any alternative in place.**

Think about what you're asking your brain to do when you try to "just stop":

"Hey brain, from now on, when we're bored, we're going to stay bored. When we're anxious, we're going to feel the full weight of that anxiety. When we're lonely, we're going to sit in that loneliness without escape. And we're going to give up the only place where we feel truly competent, connected, and in control. Sound good?"

Your brain, quite sensibly, says, "Absolutely not."

This is why trying to quit cold turkey doesn't work. You're essentially asking yourself to endure massive discomfort and give up your primary source of fulfillment without any plan for how to meet those needs differently. That's not a sustainable strategy. That's just torture.

(And then when you inevitably fail—because you're human and humans can't sustain torture indefinitely—you blame yourself for being weak. Which makes you feel worse. Which triggers more daydreaming. See how this works?)

The research backs this up. Studies on behavioral change consistently show that abstinence-only approaches fail unless they're paired with new coping strategies and alternative sources of fulfillment (Miller & Rollnick, 2012). You can't just remove a behavior. You have to replace it with something else that meets the same needs in a healthier way.

Which is exactly what we're going to do.

What Your Daydreams Are Really Telling You

Here's the reframe I want you to walk away with: **Your maladaptive daydreaming isn't a symptom of what's wrong with you. It's a symptom of what's missing from your life.**

Those elaborate fantasies where you're a hero? They're telling you that you need more competence and mastery in your real life.

Those romantic daydreams where you're deeply connected to someone? They're telling you that you're lonely and need more genuine connection.

Those scenarios where you're famous or admired? They're telling you that you need more recognition and appreciation.

Those scenes where you finally tell someone off or make your own decisions? They're telling you that you need more autonomy and control.

Your daydreams are a *map* to your values and needs. They're showing you exactly what your life is lacking. The problem is that you've been trying to satisfy those needs in a fantasy world instead of building them into your real world.

And that's what makes the Anchor & Pivot approach different. We're not just going to teach you to interrupt the drift (though we'll do that too). We're going to help you decode what your daydreams are trying to tell you about what you really need. Then we're going to help you start building those things into your actual life.

29

Because here's the truth: **You don't need to destroy your imagination. You need to build a life that's more satisfying than your fantasies.**

When real life is genuinely fulfilling—when you're regularly experiencing competence, connection, and autonomy—the pull of the fantasy world weakens. Not because you're fighting it harder, but because you don't need it as much anymore. The cookies you were smelling? You're actually eating them now, in reality. The fantasy becomes less appealing by comparison.

That's the goal. Not a life without daydreams, but a life where the daydreams serve you instead of control you. Where you can choose to use your imagination for creative projects, problem-solving, or brief mental breaks—not as an escape hatch from a life that feels unbearable.

But to get there, you need both sides of the equation. You need the ability to interrupt the drift when it happens (the Anchor), and you need to build a real life worth staying present for (the Pivot).

Let's talk about how that works.

What You Need to Remember

Your daydreams aren't random. They're serving two crucial functions: helping you escape uncomfortable emotions and providing a sense of fulfillment that your real life isn't giving you.

The addictive loop works like this: discomfort triggers the daydream, the daydream provides immediate relief and reward, but then reality returns (often with added guilt), which creates new discomfort, which triggers more daydreaming. You're stuck in a cycle where the solution keeps creating the problem.

"Just stopping" doesn't work because it requires you to sit with discomfort and give up your primary source of fulfillment without any alternative in place. That's not a failure of willpower. That's just impossible.

Your daydreams are actually showing you what you need: competence, connection, autonomy, meaning. The problem isn't the needs. The problem is that you're trying to meet them in a way that doesn't work.

The way forward isn't to kill your imagination. It's to build a real life that's more rewarding than the fantasy. When reality starts meeting your needs, the pull of the fantasy naturally weakens.

In the next chapter, we're going to introduce the practical tools that make this possible: the Anchor (for interrupting the drift) and the Pivot (for building a life worth staying present for). It's time to stop understanding the problem and start solving it.

Chapter 3: Introducing the "Anchor" and the "Pivot"

Alright. You understand what maladaptive daydreaming is. You recognize your patterns. You know why the drift is so powerful and why "just stopping" hasn't worked. Now comes the part you've been waiting for: *What do I actually do about it?*

The answer is simpler than you might think, but it requires you to work on two fronts simultaneously. You need a way to *get out* of the fantasy when you're in it (that's the **Anchor**), and you need a reason to *stay out* once you've pulled yourself back (that's the **Pivot**).

Most approaches to fixing MD focus on one or the other. They either tell you to "be more present" without giving you tools to actually do that, or they tell you to "build a better life" without addressing the fact that you can't build anything if you keep drifting away every five minutes.

You need both. The Anchor without the Pivot is torture. The Pivot without the Anchor is impossible. Together, they create a system that actually works.

Let me show you what I mean.

The Anchor: Your "Stop" Button

Imagine you're driving a car. You're cruising along, not paying much attention, and suddenly you realize you're on the wrong road heading in the wrong direction. What's the first thing you need to do?

Stop the car.

You can't course-correct while you're still barreling down the wrong path. You have to stop first, reorient yourself, and *then* choose a new direction.

The Anchor is your brake pedal. It's the skill of noticing that you've drifted into fantasy and gently bringing your attention back to the present moment—specifically, to your physical body and your immediate surroundings.

Now, I need to be clear about something: **The Anchor is not about stopping thoughts.** You can't control what thoughts show up in your mind. Trying to force yourself not to think about something is like trying not to think about white bears—it just makes the thoughts stronger. (We talked about Wegner's research on this in the introduction.)

So we're not fighting thoughts. We're redirecting *attention*.

Think of your mind like a searchlight. Right now, that searchlight is pointed at your internal fantasy world, illuminating every detail of the story playing in your head. The Anchor teaches you how to swivel that searchlight back to external reality—the feeling of your body, the things around you, the moment you're actually in.

Why the body? Because your body exists only in the present moment. Your mind can be anywhere—the past, the future, a completely imaginary world. But your body is always *here, now*. When you bring your attention to physical sensations, you automatically anchor yourself in reality.

This is based on principles from somatic psychology and mindfulness practices, which have been shown to help with various dissociative and escapist behaviors (van der Kolk, 2014). When you focus on sensory experience—what you can feel, see, hear, smell, taste—you pull yourself out of your head and into your life.

The Anchor techniques we're going to teach you in Chapter 5 are simple, fast, and concrete. We're talking 30-second interventions. Things like:

- **The 5 Senses Check**: Name five things you can see, four things you can touch, three things you can hear, two things you can smell, one thing you can taste. This forces your attention outward.
- **Feeling Your Feet**: Focus all your attention on the sensation of your feet on the floor. Notice the pressure, the texture, the temperature. Your daydream characters don't have feet. *You* do.
- **The Hand Exercise**: Press your hands together hard and notice the sensation. Or run cold water over your hands and pay attention to how it feels. Physical sensation is an immediate anchor.
- **Breath Counting**: Count three deep breaths. Just three. Feel the air moving in and out. Notice your chest rising and falling.

These aren't complicated meditation techniques that require years of practice. These are practical interventions you can use *in the moment* when you catch yourself drifting.

But here's the thing: **the Anchor alone isn't enough.** Yes, you can use these techniques to pull yourself back to reality. But if reality still feels boring, empty, or overwhelming, you're just going to drift right back into fantasy the moment you stop actively anchoring. It's like stopping the car but having nowhere to go, so you just put it back in drive and continue down the wrong road.

That's where the Pivot comes in.

The Pivot: Your "Go" Button

Let's go back to the driving metaphor. You've stopped the car. You've realized you're going the wrong direction. Now what?

You need to know where you *actually want to go*. And then you need to start driving toward that destination.

The Pivot is about building a real life that's so meaningful, so aligned with what matters to you, so genuinely fulfilling that the fantasy world starts losing its appeal. It's not about forcing yourself to stay present through sheer willpower. It's about creating a life where **you *want* to be present because there's something worth being present for**.

This is where Acceptance and Commitment Therapy (ACT) comes in, and it's going to change everything.

ACT is based on a simple but powerful idea: human suffering largely comes from trying to avoid pain and getting tangled up in unhelpful thoughts. The solution isn't to fight those thoughts or suppress that pain. The solution is to accept that discomfort is part of life, get some distance from your thoughts so they don't control you, and commit to action based on your values—the things that truly matter to you (Hayes, Strosahl, & Wilson, 2012).

Let me break down what this means for maladaptive daydreaming.

Defusion: This is the skill of seeing your daydreams as *stories your mind is telling you*, not commands you have to obey. Right now, when your mind presents a fantasy, you immediately jump into it. You fuse with it. Defusion teaches you to step back and observe: "Ah, my mind is offering me the 'hero saves the day' story again. Interesting." You're not fighting it. You're just noticing it and choosing not to engage. (We'll work on this in Chapter 6.)

Values: This is the big one. **Your daydreams are trying to tell you what you value.** If you daydream about being competent, your value is probably mastery or contribution. If you daydream about deep relationships, your value is probably connection or intimacy. If you daydream about freedom, your value is probably autonomy or self-expression. The Pivot helps you identify your core values—not what you think you *should* value, but what you *actually* care about deeply. (Chapter 7 is entirely dedicated to this.)

Committed Action: Once you know your values, you take small, concrete steps in the direction of those values in your *real life*. If connection is a value, you reach out to a friend. If competence is a value, you practice a skill. If autonomy is a value, you make a decision that's truly yours. These actions don't have to be big. They just have to be real. (We'll build your action plan in Chapter 8.)

Here's what makes the Pivot so powerful: **it directly addresses the needs your daydreams are trying to meet.** Instead of getting a fake hit of connection in your fantasy, you get real connection in your life. Instead of imagining success, you experience small, real victories. Instead of escaping from reality, you start building a reality you don't need to escape from.

And when you do that consistently, something interesting happens. The daydreams start to matter less. Not because you're fighting them harder, but because you're getting what you need from real life now. The fantasy is still there, available if you want it, but the desperate, compulsive pull weakens.

It's like when you're starving and someone puts a picture of food in front of you. That picture is intensely appealing when you're hungry. But if you've just eaten a satisfying meal? The picture is still there, but you're not obsessed with it anymore. You don't need it the same way.

That's what the Pivot does. It starts feeding you for real, so the picture (the fantasy) loses its desperate appeal.

Why You Need Both

Here's the crucial insight that a lot of approaches to MD miss: **you can't solve this problem from one direction.**

If you only work on the Anchor—learning to notice the drift and pull yourself back—you'll spend all day fighting against the pull of fantasy. It'll be exhausting. You'll constantly be resisting the urge to drift. Some days you'll succeed. Many days you won't. And even when you do succeed, you're just white-knuckling your way through a life that still doesn't feel satisfying. That's not sustainable. That's just a different kind of suffering.

On the flip side, if you only work on the Pivot—trying to build a more meaningful life—you won't be able to focus long enough to actually build anything. You'll set goals, make plans, start projects... and then drift into fantasy before you can make any real progress. You'll have great intentions and zero follow-through. (Sound familiar?)

The Anchor gets you out of the fantasy. The Pivot gives you somewhere to go.

Think of it like this: You're in a boat that's drifting away from shore. The Anchor is what stops the drift. It keeps you from floating further out to sea. But an anchor alone doesn't get you back to land. It just keeps you in one place. The Pivot is the oar that lets you row back to shore. But you can't row effectively if the boat is still drifting. You need to drop the anchor *and* start rowing.

Or here's another way to think about it: The Anchor is your defense. The Pivot is your offense. Defense stops you from losing ground. Offense moves you forward. You need both to win.

ACT research consistently shows that trying to suppress or avoid uncomfortable thoughts and urges doesn't work long-term (Hayes et al., 2012). What does work is learning to tolerate discomfort (that's the Anchor—sitting with the urge to drift without acting on it), while simultaneously building a life based on what matters (that's the Pivot—taking action toward your values).

How This Is Going to Work

Over the next six chapters, we're going to build your Anchor & Pivot toolkit step by step. Here's the roadmap:

Steps 1-2 (Chapters 4-5): Building Your Anchor

- Step 1 is about developing *awareness*. You'll learn how to notice when you're drifting, or even better, when you're *about* to drift. This is the foundation. You can't change what you don't notice.
- Step 2 is about the physical techniques that pull you back to the present moment. You'll build a personalized menu of Anchor exercises that work for your specific triggers.

Steps 3-5 (Chapters 6-8): Building Your Pivot

- Step 3 teaches you *defusion*—how to unhook from the stories your mind tells you. You'll learn to see daydreams as mental events, not commands.
- Step 4 is the most important chapter in the book. You'll decode what your daydreams are really trying to tell you about your values. This is where everything clicks into place.

- Step 5 is where you start taking action. Small, concrete steps toward your values in real life. This is what makes your actual life more compelling than fantasy.

Step 6 (Chapter 9): Harnessing Your Creativity

- You'll learn how to schedule and channel your imaginative capacity into productive creative work. We're not killing your daydreaming. We're teaching you to use it on purpose.

Then in Part 3, we'll talk about what to do when you relapse (because you will—everyone does), and what life looks like when you're in control of the drift instead of the other way around.

Each chapter will have exercises and worksheets. You'll need to actually do them. Reading about these tools won't help if you don't practice them. But I promise, they're short and practical. No hour-long meditations or complicated journaling protocols. Just simple actions you can take right now.

The Mindset Shift You Need to Make

Before we jump into the practical tools, there's one more thing you need to understand. This isn't about achieving perfection. This isn't about never daydreaming again. This isn't even about "curing" yourself.

This is about taking back control.

You're going to drift sometimes. That's fine. You're human. But instead of being dragged into fantasy against your will, spending hours there, and then feeling awful about it, you're going to learn how to notice it's happening, pull yourself back, understand what need you were trying to meet, and take a real-world action toward that need.

Sometimes you're going to consciously choose to daydream—maybe you're using that time for creative work, or you're deliberately giving yourself a mental break, or you're exploring an idea for a story you want to write. That's different. That's using your imagination intentionally. That's not MD. That's just being a creative person.

The difference is *choice*. Right now, you don't have a choice. The drift happens automatically, and you can't stop it even when you want to. The goal is to give you back that choice. To make you the one in charge, not your fantasies.

And here's what's great: as you practice the Anchor & Pivot skills, that control gets easier. The neural pathways that currently connect "uncomfortable feeling" to "initiate daydream" start to weaken. New pathways form: "uncomfortable feeling" to "notice and anchor" to "take values-based action." Your brain rewires itself through practice.

Neuroscience calls this *neuroplasticity*—the brain's ability to form new connections and patterns throughout life (Doidge, 2007). You're not stuck with the patterns you have now. You can build new ones. But it takes practice and repetition.

So yeah, this is going to take work. But it's not impossible work. It's totally doable work. And every time you successfully notice the drift, anchor yourself, and pivot toward something meaningful in real life? You're rewiring your brain just a little bit more.

Over time, those little changes add up to a completely different relationship with your imagination.

A relationship where *you're* in the driver's seat.

The Foundation Is Set

You now have the framework that's going to guide everything else in this book. The Anchor stops the drift by pulling your attention to your body and the present moment. The Pivot builds a life worth staying present for by connecting you to your values and helping you take meaningful action.

You need both. Defense and offense. Stop and go. Awareness and action.

The Anchor alone is just resistance—exhausting and ultimately unsustainable. The Pivot alone is just good intentions that never get implemented because you keep drifting before you can follow through.

Together, they create a system that actually works. You interrupt the pattern (Anchor) while simultaneously building something better (Pivot). You're not just fighting against the fantasy. You're actively creating a reality that's more satisfying.

In the next chapter, we start building the first Anchor skill: noticing the drift before it carries you away. You can't change what you can't see. So let's learn how to see it clearly.

Chapter 4: Notice the Drift (The "Anchor" Skill 1)

Jessica is 28. She works in marketing. Every morning, she sits down at her computer with her coffee, opens her email, and tells herself, "Today's the day. I'm going to stay focused."

Five minutes later, she's somewhere else. Not in the office. Not at her desk. She's accepting an award for best campaign of the year. The applause is thunderous. Her boss—who barely acknowledges her in real life—is beaming with pride. She's giving a speech. It's eloquent and funny, and everyone is hanging on every word.

Twenty minutes pass before she notices what's happening. The email is still unread. The coffee is still untouched. And that familiar sinking feeling hits her stomach.

"I did it again."

But here's the question: when did "again" actually start? Was it when she opened her email? When she sat down at her desk? When she woke up this morning already thinking about the fantasy? Or was it even earlier—last night when she set up tomorrow's drift by mentally planning which scenes she'd revisit?

The drift doesn't start when you notice it. It starts well before that.

And this is why the first Anchor skill isn't about pulling yourself back from daydreaming. It's about learning to catch yourself *earlier in the process*—ideally before you're fully immersed, but at minimum, while you still have some awareness that it's happening.

This skill is called *meta-awareness*, and it's the foundation for everything else we're going to do. You can't anchor yourself if you don't know you're drifting. You can't change a pattern you don't notice. So let's learn how to see it clearly.

What Meta-Awareness Actually Means

Meta-awareness sounds fancy, but it's simple: **it's the ability to know what your mind is doing while it's doing it.**

Right now, you're reading these words. But are you *aware* that you're reading? Or are you on autopilot, eyes moving across the page while your mind is half-planning what you'll eat for dinner? Meta-awareness is that moment when you step back and think, "Oh, I'm reading right now. And actually, I'm not really paying attention. I should focus."

For people with maladaptive daydreaming, meta-awareness is the moment when you realize, "Wait. I'm not working on this document. I'm in my head, running through that fantasy scene. I've been here for... how long?"

Research on mind-wandering shows that most people spend nearly half their waking hours with their minds somewhere other than the present moment (Schooler et al., 2011). But here's what's interesting: there are two types of mind-wandering. There's *tuned-out* mind-wandering, where you have no idea your mind has drifted until something external snaps you back (like someone calling your name). And there's *tuned-in* mind-wandering, where you catch yourself in the act—you notice that you've drifted and you can choose to redirect your attention (Smallwood & Schooler, 2006).

The difference between these two types? Meta-awareness.

People who regularly practice meta-awareness catch themselves drifting more quickly. They spend less time lost in unproductive thought. They have more control over where their attention goes. And this is exactly what you need to develop.

But here's the thing: **meta-awareness isn't about judging yourself.** This is crucial. If every time you notice you're daydreaming, you immediately think, "God, I'm doing it again, I'm so pathetic, why can't I stop this?"—you're going to start avoiding the awareness itself. Your brain will learn that noticing equals pain, so it'll stop letting you notice. You'll stay tuned-out because tuning-in feels awful.

We need to separate the *noticing* from the *judging*.

Noticing is just information: "Oh, I'm daydreaming right now." That's it. Neutral. Factual. Like noticing, "Oh, it's raining" or "Oh, I'm hungry." There's no moral weight to the observation. You're just becoming aware of what's happening.

The judging comes after: "I'm such a failure. I'll never change. This is hopeless." That's the part we're going to let go of. Because judgment doesn't help you change. It just makes you feel terrible, which—guess what?—triggers more daydreaming as an escape from the terrible feeling.

So meta-awareness, done right, is *kind*. It's curious. It's interested. "Huh, I'm drifting again. Interesting. What triggered that? What was I feeling right before I drifted?"

This is the mindset we're building. Awareness without judgment. Noticing without shame.

The Early Warning System

Most people with MD only notice they're daydreaming after they've been deep in it for a while. They "wake up" from the fantasy and realize significant time has passed. By then, it's hard to pull back. The fantasy has momentum. The neural pathway is fully activated. You're so immersed that redirecting feels almost impossible.

So we need to catch it earlier. **Way earlier.**

Think of it like a fire. Once a building is fully engulfed in flames, putting it out is a massive effort requiring professional firefighters and huge amounts of resources. But if you notice the *spark* before it spreads? You can stamp it out with your foot.

Your daydreaming follows the same pattern. There's a progression:

The Setup → The Trigger → The Drift Begins → Full Immersion → The "Snap Back"

Right now, you're probably only catching yourself at the "Full Immersion" or "Snap Back" stages. We're going to train you to notice at "The Setup" or "The Trigger" stage. Because that's where you have the most power to redirect.

So what does "The Setup" look like?

Michael, a 35-year-old teacher, describes it this way: "I realize now that I set up my daydreaming sessions in advance without even knowing it. I'll be finishing dinner, and I'll think, 'After I clean up, I'll go to my room and just relax for a bit.' But 'relax' is code. What I really mean is 'daydream for three hours.' I'm already planning it. I'm already looking forward to it. The drift starts way before I actually lie down on my bed and put on music."

45

The setup is subtle. It's the thought, "I'll just put on this playlist while I work." (You know that playlist always triggers you.) It's opening a blank document "to brainstorm ideas" when you're really creating a space to mentally drift. It's deciding to take a walk "to clear your head" when what you're really doing is giving yourself permission to pace and fantasize.

You're setting up the drift before it happens. And if you can catch yourself during the setup, you can make a different choice.

Identifying Your Personal Warning Signs

Every person has specific warning signs that they're about to drift or are in the early stages of drifting. These are like the smoke before the fire. If you learn to recognize your smoke signals, you can intervene before you're fully engulfed.

Common warning signs include:

Physical movements:

- Reaching for headphones or earbuds
- Starting to pace back and forth
- Getting into a specific position (lying on your bed a certain way, sitting in a particular chair)
- Fidgeting or repetitive movements (twirling hair, tapping fingers, rocking)

Environmental changes:

- Closing the door to your room
- Dimming the lights
- Putting on specific music
- Positioning yourself so no one can see your screen

Mental shifts:

- A sudden urge to be alone
- Feeling restless or bored and looking for an "escape"
- Thinking about your fantasy characters or plotlines even though you're supposed to be focusing on something else
- A sense of anticipation building—like you're looking forward to something, and that something is the drift

Emotional triggers:

- Feeling stressed, anxious, or overwhelmed
- Feeling lonely or disconnected
- Feeling inadequate after a failure or comparison
- Feeling bored with no clear task to engage with

Here's what's fascinating: once you start paying attention, you'll discover that your drift follows a pattern. It's not random. The same sequence of events happens almost every time. For you, it might be: feel stressed → put on music → start pacing → drift begins within two minutes. For someone else, it might be: finish task → feel bored → open social media → see something that reminds them of their fantasy → drift begins.

Your job is to identify your specific pattern.

And the earlier in the sequence you can catch yourself, the easier it is to redirect. Catching yourself as you reach for headphones? Much easier to stop than catching yourself 30 minutes into a full fantasy scene.

Exercise: The Trigger Tracker

Alright, time to get scientific about your own brain. For the next week, you're going to track your daydreaming sessions. Not to judge yourself. Not to feel bad about how many there are. Just to gather data about your patterns.

You're going to need a notebook, your phone's notes app, or a simple spreadsheet. Every time you catch yourself daydreaming—at any stage—you're going to log the following information:

1. Date and Time When did this happen? What time of day?

2. Location Where were you? (At your desk, in bed, in your car, walking outside, etc.)

3. What You Were Supposed to Be Doing What task were you avoiding or distracted from?

4. The Trigger (if you can identify it) What happened right before you started drifting?

- Did you put on music? Which song or playlist?
- Did you start a repetitive movement?
- Were you feeling a specific emotion?
- Did something remind you of your fantasy?
- Did you deliberately set up the drift?

5. How You Felt Right Before What was your emotional state? Bored? Anxious? Lonely? Frustrated? Overwhelmed? Fine but understimulated?

6. The Plot/Theme What were you daydreaming about? (Use shorthand—"the hero plot," "the romance scenario," "the confrontation scene," etc.)

7. How Long You Think You Were Gone Your best estimate. (You might not know exactly, but take a guess.)

8. How You Noticed Did you catch yourself during the drift? Did something external snap you out of it? Did you not even realize until much later?

Here's an example entry:

Date/Time: Tuesday, 2:30 PM
Location: My desk at work
Task I Was Avoiding: Quarterly report
Trigger: Opened a blank document to "outline" the report. Felt overwhelmed by how much work it would take.
Emotion Before: Stressed, inadequate
Plot: The "successful professional" plot—presenting my work to executives who are impressed
Duration: About 25 minutes
How I Noticed: Coworker asked me a question and I snapped back

Do this for a week. **Every single time you catch yourself.** Even if it's ten times a day. (No judgment, just data.)

At the end of the week, look for patterns:

- **Time patterns**: Are you more likely to drift in the morning? Afternoon? Evening? When you first sit down to work? Right before bed?
- **Location patterns**: Does it always happen in certain places? Your room? Your car? Specific chair?
- **Trigger patterns**: What are your top three triggers? Music? Specific emotional states? Boredom? Repetitive movements?
- **Theme patterns**: Do you have go-to fantasy plots? Do they change based on your emotional state?
- **Duration patterns**: Are some drifts longer than others? What makes the difference?

This information is gold. Because once you know your patterns, you can start to *intervene* in those patterns. You can catch yourself at the setup stage. You can recognize when you're creating conditions for a drift and make a different choice.

Building Your Meta-Awareness Muscle

Tracking your patterns is step one. But we also need to strengthen your ability to notice in real-time. This requires practice, just like building physical strength requires exercise.

Here are three techniques to develop stronger meta-awareness:

Technique 1: The Hourly Check-In

Set a gentle alarm on your phone to go off once an hour during your waking hours. (Make it a pleasant sound, not a jarring one.) When it goes off, pause whatever you're doing and ask yourself:

"What am I doing right now? Am I present, or am I somewhere else mentally?"

That's it. Just check in. If you're present—great, go back to what you were doing. If you're drifting or starting to drift—you've just caught it. Notice it without judgment, and then decide what to do next. (We'll get to the "what to do next" part in Chapter 5.)

Research on mindfulness practices shows that regular check-ins throughout the day significantly improve people's ability to catch mind-wandering early (Brewer et al., 2011). The alarm isn't meant to interrupt you forever. It's training wheels. After a few weeks of hourly check-ins, your brain gets better at checking in automatically.

Technique 2: The Trigger Alert

Based on your Trigger Tracker data, identify your top three triggers. Let's say yours are: (1) putting on music, (2) feeling stressed, and (3) being alone in your room.

For each trigger, create a mental "alert." This is like a popup notification in your mind. The moment you notice the trigger happening, you think:

"Alert: This is a trigger. I'm about to drift. Do I want to?"

Again, no judgment. Just awareness. You're giving yourself the chance to choose instead of operating on autopilot. Sometimes you'll decide, "Yes, I actually have 20 minutes and I'm going to intentionally daydream right now." (That's fine—we'll talk about intentional daydreaming in Chapter 9.) But most of the time, you'll recognize, "No, I'm using this as an escape from something uncomfortable. I should stay present."

The key is catching the trigger as it's happening, not 20 minutes later.

Technique 3: The Mental Label

This technique comes from mindfulness meditation, and it's incredibly simple. Whenever you notice your mind wandering— even slightly—you label it. Just think the word "thinking" or "drifting" or "fantasy." You don't have to say it out loud. Just acknowledge it mentally.

"Thinking."

Then gently redirect your attention back to whatever you're supposed to be doing. If your mind wanders again five seconds later (which it probably will), you label it again. "Thinking." And redirect again.

This isn't about getting frustrated that your mind keeps wandering. That's normal. Minds wander constantly. The practice is in the *noticing* and the *redirecting*. Each time you notice and redirect, you're strengthening the meta-awareness pathway in your brain. You're literally building new neural connections that support awareness (Tang et al., 2015).

Do this for just five minutes a day while working on a task. Set a timer. Every time your mind drifts, label it and come back. You'll probably label it dozens of times in five minutes. That's perfect. That's the practice.

What to Do When You Notice (Preview)

You might be wondering: "Okay, so I notice I'm drifting. Then what?"

That's exactly what Chapter 5 is about—the physical anchoring techniques that pull you back to the present moment. But for now, just focus on building the noticing muscle. Because you can't use any anchoring technique if you don't first recognize that you need to use it.

For this week, your only job is to notice. Track your patterns. Check in hourly. Create trigger alerts. Label your thoughts when they wander.

Don't try to stop the daydreaming yet. (I know that sounds counterintuitive, but trust me on this.) Just practice noticing without judgment. Get really good at catching yourself, especially in the early stages before you're fully immersed.

Think of this week as reconnaissance. You're a scientist studying your own behavior. You're gathering intelligence about how your particular brain works. This information is going to make everything else we do much more effective.

The Power of Noticing Without Doing

Here's something that might surprise you: **just by practicing meta-awareness, your daydreaming will probably start to decrease on its own.**

Research on behavior change shows that simply monitoring a behavior makes people do it less, even without any other intervention (Burke et al., 2011). This is called *self-monitoring*, and it works because awareness itself disrupts automatic patterns. When you're operating on autopilot, behaviors flow smoothly without any conscious thought. But the moment you start paying attention, you introduce a tiny pause—a gap between trigger and response. And in that gap, change becomes possible.

So don't underestimate the power of what you're doing this week. Tracking your triggers, checking in hourly, labeling your thoughts—these aren't just preparatory exercises. They're already starting to change your relationship with daydreaming.

You're moving from being controlled by the drift to being aware of the drift. That's huge.

And awareness, practiced consistently, builds the foundation for control.

What You're Taking With You

Meta-awareness is the ability to notice what your mind is doing while it's doing it. It's awareness without judgment—just neutral, curious observation of your mental state.

You can't change a pattern you don't notice, so the first step is learning to catch yourself drifting. The earlier you catch it— ideally at the "setup" or "trigger" stage—the easier it is to redirect.

53

Your daydreaming follows a pattern. By tracking your sessions for a week using the Trigger Tracker, you'll identify your specific triggers, common themes, timing patterns, and warning signs. This information is essential for everything that follows.

Building meta-awareness requires practice. Use hourly check-ins, trigger alerts, and mental labeling to strengthen your noticing muscle. The more you practice, the faster you'll catch yourself.

Just by paying attention to your daydreaming patterns, you'll likely start to do it less. Awareness itself disrupts automatic behaviors. You're already creating change just by noticing.

In the next chapter, we'll learn what to do once you've noticed you're drifting: the physical anchoring techniques that bring you back to the present moment in 30 seconds or less. But first, spend this week practicing the noticing. Get really good at catching yourself. Everything else builds on this foundation.

Chapter 5: Drop the Anchor (The "Anchor" Skill 2)

You've noticed. That's the first victory. You caught yourself drifting—maybe while you were still reaching for your headphones, maybe five minutes into a fantasy scene, maybe somewhere in between. The awareness is there. You know what's happening.

Now what?

This is the moment where most people try to "think" their way out. They tell themselves, "Stop it. Focus. Come on, be present." They try to force their mind back to the task at hand through sheer mental willpower.

And it doesn't work.

Because you can't think your way out of a mental drift. You can't use your mind to fix a mind problem. That's like trying to fix a flooded basement by dumping more water into it. You need a different tool.

You need your body.

Your body is the most reliable anchor you have. While your mind can be anywhere—lost in fantasy, obsessing about the past, worrying about the future—your body is always here, always now. You can't physically daydream. Your body doesn't travel to imaginary places. It stays planted in reality, waiting for you to pay attention to it.

This is why somatic (body-based) techniques are so effective for pulling yourself back from dissociation, rumination, and yes, maladaptive daydreaming (Ogden et al., 2006). When you shift your attention from your thoughts to your physical sensations, you automatically land in the present moment.

And the best part? **These techniques take 30 seconds or less.**

We're not talking about hour-long body scans or complex yoga routines. We're talking about quick, simple interventions that you can do anywhere, anytime, without anyone even noticing.

Let's learn how to drop the anchor.

Why Physical Sensation Works

Here's what's happening in your brain when you're deep in a daydream. Your prefrontal cortex—the part responsible for executive function and directed attention—is essentially offline. Your default mode network—the part that handles internal thought, imagination, and self-referential processing—is running the show (Buckner et al., 2008). You're internally focused. The external world fades into the background.

To snap out of this state, you need to activate different neural circuits. Specifically, you need to engage the parts of your brain that process sensory information from the outside world and from your body. When you focus on physical sensations, you switch neural gears. The default mode network quiets down, and the sensory processing regions light up.

This isn't magic. It's just neuroscience. **Your brain can't fully attend to both internal fantasy and external sensation at the same time.** Sure, you can switch back and forth rapidly, but you can't do both simultaneously. So when you deliberately focus on the feeling of your feet on the floor or the sensation of cold water on your hands, you're essentially hijacking your brain's attention system and redirecting it to reality.

Research on grounding techniques—which are essentially what we're teaching here—shows they're highly effective for interrupting dissociative states and bringing people back to the present moment (Najavits, 2001). And maladaptive daydreaming, while not exactly the same as dissociation, operates on similar principles. You're mentally elsewhere, disconnected from your immediate reality. Grounding brings you back.

The key is to make these techniques so simple and so quick that you'll actually use them. Because the perfect technique that you never use is useless. We need techniques that are practical, accessible, and effective in the moment.

The Core Anchoring Techniques

Here are five powerful anchoring techniques. You don't need to use all of them. Try each one and see which ones resonate with you. Then those become your go-to tools.

Technique 1: The 5-4-3-2-1 Sensory Check

This is one of the most reliable grounding techniques, and it works by forcing your attention through all five senses (Bourne, 2015).

When you notice you're drifting, pause and do this:

- **See 5 things**: Name five things you can see right now. Look around and actually identify them. "Desk. Coffee mug. Window. That crack in the wall. My phone."
- **Touch 4 things**: Notice four things you can feel. "The chair against my back. My feet on the floor. The pen in my hand. The texture of my jeans."
- **Hear 3 things**: Identify three sounds. "The hum of the air conditioner. Someone talking down the hall. The tapping of my fingers on the desk."

- **Smell 2 things**: Notice two things you can smell. This one's harder, so sometimes you have to really pay attention. "The coffee. A faint smell of... dust? Or maybe just air."
- **Taste 1 thing**: What can you taste? Even if it's just the taste of your mouth. "The mint from the gum I had earlier."

By the time you've worked through all five senses, you're back. Your attention is fully external, anchored in your immediate environment. The fantasy is still there as a memory, but you're not immersed in it anymore.

This takes about 30-45 seconds. That's it.

Technique 2: Feel Your Feet

This one is almost embarrassingly simple, but it works.

Bring all your attention to your feet. Notice how they feel right now. Are they pressed against the floor? In shoes or barefoot? Warm or cold? Can you feel each toe? The arch of your foot? The heel?

Really pay attention. Wiggle your toes if that helps. Press your feet into the floor and notice the pressure. Focus only on the physical sensations in your feet for 15-20 seconds.

Your fantasy characters don't have feet. They don't have weight or physical presence. You do. And when you focus on that physical presence, you can't simultaneously be lost in imaginary space.

This technique is especially useful in meetings or situations where you need to stay present but you've started to drift. No one can tell you're doing it. You just quietly refocus on your feet, and within seconds, you're back.

Technique 3: Cold Water on Hands

This one requires access to a sink, but it's incredibly effective because the temperature creates such a strong sensory signal.

When you realize you're drifting, get up and go to the nearest bathroom or kitchen. Run cold water over your hands. Really cold if you can stand it. Hold them under the stream and pay complete attention to how it feels.

Notice the temperature. Notice the pressure of the water. Notice how your hands feel different when you move them closer or further from the faucet. Keep your full attention on the sensation for 20-30 seconds.

The coldness is a powerful interrupt signal. It's hard to stay lost in fantasy when your hands are under freezing water. Your brain immediately orients to the physical sensation because it's strong and mildly uncomfortable. (That's why it works.)

Technique 4: The Hand Press

This one you can do anywhere, anytime, without anyone noticing. It's perfect for situations where you can't get up or make any obvious movements.

Press your hands together in front of you, palm to palm, like you're praying. Press them together hard. Really hard. Feel the pressure. Feel the warmth building between your palms. Notice the sensation in your fingers, your wrists, your forearms.

Hold for 10-15 seconds, pressing as hard as you comfortably can. Then release and notice how your hands feel. That tingling sensation? That's you, back in your body.

Alternatively, you can press one hand against your thigh under the table, or press your palms down on your desk. The key is the physical pressure and the attention you give to that sensation.

Technique 5: Breath Counting

This is the only technique that uses breath, and we're keeping it simple. No fancy breathing patterns. Just counting.

When you notice you're drifting, bring your attention to your breath. You don't have to change how you're breathing. Just notice it. Then count three breaths.

Breath one: Feel the air coming in through your nose, filling your lungs, then leaving your body.
Breath two: Notice your chest or belly rising and falling.
Breath three: Pay attention to the temperature of the air—cool on the way in, warm on the way out.

Three breaths. That's all. Somewhere between 15 and 30 seconds depending on how fast you breathe.

Breath is always available, always with you, and focusing on it brings you immediately into the present. You can't breathe in the past or the future. You can only breathe now. So when you pay attention to your breath, you're automatically present.

This Isn't About Stopping Thoughts

Let me be really clear about something: **these techniques don't stop your thoughts. They redirect your attention.**

Your mind might still be offering you the fantasy. The story might still be there, playing in the background like a movie you've paused but can keep hearing from the other room. That's fine. We're not trying to make thoughts disappear.

We're just moving the spotlight of your attention from internal fantasy to external and physical reality.

Think of it like this: Your daydream is a radio station that your mind can tune into. Right now, that station is playing loudly, and you're completely absorbed in it. The anchoring techniques don't destroy the station. They just switch the channel. They retune your attention to the "Present Moment" station—the one broadcasting sensations from your body and your environment.

The fantasy station might still be there in the background, especially at first. But by focusing on your feet or your breath or the cold water on your hands, you're choosing a different channel. You're choosing reality.

And the more often you practice switching channels, the easier it gets. The neural pathway from "notice drift" to "anchor in body" gets stronger. Eventually, it becomes almost automatic. You notice, you anchor, you're back. Five seconds flat.

But only if you practice. Which brings us to your assignment.

Creating Your Personal Anchor Menu

Different triggers call for different anchoring techniques. The technique that works perfectly when you're alone at home might not work when you're in a meeting. The technique that works when you're bored might not work when you're anxious.

So you need a menu of options—different techniques for different situations.

Here's how to build yours:

Step 1: Review Your Trigger Tracker

Look at the patterns you identified in Chapter 4. What are your top three triggers? For most people, they'll be things like:

- Specific music or sounds
- Being alone in a certain location (bedroom, car, etc.)
- Feeling a particular emotion (stress, boredom, loneliness)
- Specific movements (pacing, lying down a certain way)

Write down your top three triggers.

Step 2: Match Anchors to Triggers

For each trigger, ask yourself: "Which anchoring technique would be most practical and effective in this situation?"

Let's say your trigger is "putting on music while working at my desk." In that situation, the Hand Press or Feel Your Feet techniques would work well because you can do them right there without getting up. The 5-4-3-2-1 would also work.

But if your trigger is "feeling anxious before a social event," the Cold Water on Hands technique might be perfect because you can excuse yourself to the bathroom and do it.

If your trigger is "lying in bed at night," Breath Counting or Feel Your Feet would work because you can do them lying down.

Match at least two anchoring techniques to each of your triggers. This gives you options.

Step 3: Write It Down

Actually write out your Anchor Menu. It might look something like this:

MY ANCHOR MENU

Trigger 1: Putting on music at my desk

- Primary Anchor: Feel Your Feet
- Backup Anchor: Hand Press

Trigger 2: Feeling stressed about a work task

- Primary Anchor: Cold Water on Hands (go to bathroom)
- Backup Anchor: 5-4-3-2-1 Sensory Check

Trigger 3: Being alone in my room at night

- Primary Anchor: Breath Counting
- Backup Anchor: Feel Your Feet

Put this somewhere you can see it. On your phone. On a sticky note on your computer. In your wallet. The point is to have a plan *before* the trigger happens, so you're not trying to figure out what to do in the moment when you're already starting to drift.

Practice Makes It Automatic

Here's the truth: these techniques will feel awkward the first few times you use them. They might not even seem to "work" immediately. That's normal. You're building a new skill, and new skills always feel clunky at first.

But if you practice them consistently—every time you notice you're drifting—they'll become second nature. The awkwardness fades. The effectiveness increases. And eventually, the process becomes: notice drift → anchor → back to present. Boom. Done in 30 seconds.

Here's how to practice:

Practice Schedule (This Week)

- **At least 3 times a day**, intentionally practice one of your anchoring techniques. Set a reminder on your phone if needed. You don't even have to be drifting. Just practice the physical motion of anchoring so your body and brain learn the pattern.
- **Every time you catch yourself drifting** (even a little bit), use one of your techniques immediately. Don't think about it. Don't wait. Just drop the anchor as soon as you notice.
- **At the end of each day**, jot down a quick note: How many times did you drift today? How many times did you use an anchor? Which technique worked best?

You're building a habit loop: **Notice → Anchor → Redirect.** The more you practice this loop, the more automatic it becomes.

And here's what's going to happen: You'll start catching yourself earlier in the drift process. Your meta-awareness from Chapter 4 is growing stronger, and now you have a practical tool to use the moment you notice. So instead of drifting for 30 minutes before you catch yourself, you'll drift for 5 minutes. Then 2 minutes. Then you'll catch yourself as you're reaching for your headphones, and you'll anchor before you even start.

That's the goal. Not perfection. Not never drifting. Just catching it faster and pulling yourself back more easily.

What If It Doesn't Work?

Sometimes you'll use an anchoring technique and it won't feel like it's working. You'll do the 5-4-3-2-1, and part of your mind is still in the fantasy. Or you'll focus on your feet, and within 10 seconds you're drifting back.

This is normal, especially at first. A few reasons this might happen:

You're already too deep in the drift: If you've been immersed in fantasy for 20+ minutes, the momentum is strong. You might need to use an anchoring technique multiple times, or string two techniques together. Do Feel Your Feet, then immediately do Breath Counting. The combination might be what you need.

The emotional trigger is still active: If you're anxious or stressed, and that's what triggered the drift, anchoring will bring you back to... being anxious and stressed. Which immediately makes you want to drift again. In this case, the anchor gets you back, but then you need the Pivot (which we'll learn in the next chapters) to address the underlying emotional need. For now, just know that sometimes you'll need to re-anchor multiple times until the trigger emotion settles.

You're fighting the technique: Some people try to anchor while simultaneously resisting it. They're doing the technique but also thinking, "This is stupid, this won't work, I should just give up." That internal resistance makes it harder. Try to bring curiosity instead of skepticism. Just try it sincerely for one week and see what happens.

You need a different technique: Not every technique works for every person. If one isn't working, try another. That's why you have a menu.

And here's the most important thing: **even if the anchor only brings you back for 30 seconds before you drift again, that's still a win.** You practiced the skill. You redirected your attention, even briefly. That's progress. Do it again. And again. Each time, you're strengthening the neural pathway.

This isn't about perfection. It's about practice.

Bringing It All Together

The anchor is your stop button—your way of interrupting the drift and bringing yourself back to the present moment by focusing on physical sensation. Your body is always here, always now, and when you pay attention to it, you can't simultaneously be lost in fantasy.

The five core anchoring techniques are: 5-4-3-2-1 Sensory Check, Feel Your Feet, Cold Water on Hands, The Hand Press, and Breath Counting. Each takes 30 seconds or less. Try them all and find which ones work best for you.

These techniques don't stop thoughts—they redirect attention. You're switching channels from internal fantasy to external reality. The fantasy might still be there in the background, but you're no longer absorbed in it.

Create your personal Anchor Menu by matching specific techniques to your specific triggers. Write it down so you have a plan before the drift happens.

Practice these techniques at least three times a day this week, plus every time you catch yourself drifting. The more you practice, the more automatic the Notice → Anchor → Redirect loop becomes.

The anchor brings you back, but it doesn't answer the question: back to what? That's where the Pivot comes in. In the next three chapters, we're going to build a real life that's actually worth staying present for—a life that's more compelling than your fantasies.

Chapter 6: Unhook from the Story (The "Pivot" Skill 1: Defusion)

You've just used an anchoring technique. You felt your feet on the floor, counted three breaths, maybe ran cold water over your hands. You're back. Present. Grounded in your body and the here and now.

But your mind? **Your mind is still talking.**

"Just five minutes in the fantasy won't hurt. You've been working hard. You deserve a break. Besides, you were at such a good part of the story. The hero was about to finally get the recognition they deserved, and—actually, wait, what if instead of that scene, we go back to the earlier one and change how the confrontation happens? That would be so much better. We could replay it with different dialogue..."

And just like that, if you're not careful, you're drifting again.

Because here's the thing about your mind: **it's a story-making machine, and it's really good at its job.** It's constantly generating narratives, creating scenarios, offering you mental movies to watch. That's normal. That's what minds do. The problem isn't that your mind offers you these stories. The problem is that you've been treating those stories as commands you have to follow.

Your mind says, "Let's daydream about being a hero," and you immediately obey. Your mind says, "Let's replay that fantasy relationship scene," and you drop everything to do it. You've fused with the stories—you've merged with them so completely that you can't tell the difference between "my mind is offering me a thought" and "I need to act on this thought right now."

This chapter is about learning to unhook.

It's about seeing your daydreams for what they are: mental events, stories your brain is generating, movies your mind wants to show you—but not commands you have to obey. When you can create that distance, when you can observe the stories without immediately jumping into them, everything changes.

This is called *cognitive defusion*, and it's one of the most powerful skills from Acceptance and Commitment Therapy (Harris, 2009).

What Fusion Looks Like

Let's say you're working on a project. It's tedious. Your mind starts to wander. And then a thought appears: "Wouldn't it be better to imagine that scenario where you finally stand up to your boss?"

Right now, here's what probably happens:

The thought appears → You immediately engage with it → You're in the fantasy within seconds

You've *fused* with the thought. You bought into it completely. You didn't question it or observe it. You just followed it, like a dog following a scent, straight into the fantasy world.

Fusion happens so fast that you don't even notice the transition. One moment you're working on the project, the next moment you're deep in the daydream, and you don't even remember making the decision to go there.

This is what psychologists mean by "cognitive fusion"—you're so tangled up with your thoughts that you can't separate yourself from them (Hayes et al., 2012). The thought and the action are one seamless event. No gap. No space to choose.

68

And this is a problem, because **not every thought deserves action.** Your mind generates thousands of thoughts every day. Most of them are useless. Some are actively unhelpful. If you followed every single thought your mind offered, you'd be a mess. (Imagine actually doing every weird thing your mind suggests when you're standing on a high balcony or driving on the highway. Yeah, that would end badly.)

You already practice defusion in other areas of your life without realizing it. If you're on a diet and you think, "I really want a donut," you don't necessarily eat the donut. You observe the thought, maybe feel the craving, and then decide whether to act on it or not. There's a gap between thought and action.

We need to create that same gap with your daydreaming thoughts.

What Defusion Looks Like

Defusion is simple. It's the practice of noticing thoughts *as thoughts*—as mental events that you can observe without acting on them.

Here's what the process looks like with defusion:

The thought appears → You notice it → You label it → You let it be there without engaging → You redirect to what matters

Let's break that down:

The thought appears: "Wouldn't it be better to imagine that scenario where you finally stand up to your boss?"

You notice it: "Oh, my mind is offering me a thought about daydreaming."

You label it: "There's the 'confrontation plot' again."

You let it be there without engaging: "Interesting. My mind really likes this story. I'm not going to follow it right now, but I see that it's here."

You redirect to what matters: "Back to the project."

See the difference? You didn't fight the thought. You didn't try to suppress it or force it away. You just observed it, labeled it, and chose not to act on it.

The thought is still there. Your mind might keep offering it, like a persistent salesperson. "But seriously, that confrontation scene though. Wouldn't it be good? Just five minutes." And you observe that too. "Ah, my mind is still trying to sell me on this daydream. That's what minds do."

The story can play in the background if it wants to. You're just not buying a ticket to watch it.

This is what research on ACT calls "psychological flexibility"—the ability to contact the present moment while observing your thoughts without getting hooked by them, and then choose actions based on your values instead of your momentary thoughts (Hayes et al., 2012). It's one of the strongest predictors of mental health and well-being.

And it's a skill you can learn.

Practical Defusion Techniques

Here are five techniques for unhooking from your daydream stories. Like the anchoring techniques, try them all and see which ones resonate with you.

Technique 1: Thank Your Mind

This one sounds weird, but it works. When your mind offers you a daydream, instead of fighting it or following it, just thank it.

"Thanks, mind, for that thought."

"Thanks for the suggestion, brain."

"I appreciate the offer, but I'm going to pass right now."

You're treating your mind like a helpful (if sometimes misguided) assistant that's trying to make suggestions. You're acknowledging the thought without obeying it. This creates distance and a touch of humor, which helps prevent fusion.

Research shows that thanking your mind for intrusive thoughts reduces their power and frequency over time (Masuda et al., 2004). It's counterintuitive—you'd think acknowledging the thought would make it stronger—but the opposite is true. When you stop fighting thoughts, they lose their grip.

Technique 2: Name the Story

Give your recurring daydream plots names, like you're titling movies or TV episodes.

"Oh, there's 'The Hero Saves the Day' plot again."

"Looks like 'The Perfect Romance' is playing."

"Here comes 'The Epic Confrontation,' Season 3, Episode 47."

When you name the story, you create distance. You're not *in* the story anymore. You're observing it from outside, like you're scrolling through Netflix deciding whether to watch something.

71

And just like with Netflix, you can see the title, think "Eh, not interested right now," and move on to something else. You don't have to watch every show your mind suggests.

Technique 3: Use the Phrase "I'm Having the Thought That..."

This is a classic ACT technique. Instead of thinking, "I need to escape into my fantasy right now," you reframe it as, "I'm having the thought that I need to escape into my fantasy right now."

Seems like a small change, right? But it's actually huge. The first version makes it sound like a fact, a reality, an urgent need. The second version makes it clear that it's just a thought—a mental event that your brain generated.

Try it with your daydreaming urges:

Instead of: "I want to daydream"
Reframe as: "I'm having the thought that I want to daydream"

Instead of: "I need to escape right now"
Reframe as: "I'm noticing the urge to escape right now"

Adding that little prefix—"I'm having the thought that" or "I'm noticing"—creates space between you and the urge. You're not the urge. You're the person observing the urge. Big difference.

Technique 4: Let It Play in the Background

Sometimes your mind is going to be persistent. It's going to keep offering you the daydream, keep tempting you with the fantasy. Fighting it just makes it louder.

So don't fight it. Just let it be there, like background music in a store.

"Okay, mind. You can keep playing that story if you want. I'm going to focus on this task, but you do your thing."

You're not engaging with it. You're not giving it your full attention. But you're also not trying to silence it. It's just... there. In the background. Like the hum of traffic or the sound of rain.

And here's what happens: when you stop fighting the thought, when you stop giving it all your energy through resistance, it often fades on its own. Not always immediately, but eventually. Because thoughts need attention to persist. When you stop feeding them attention, they get bored and wander off.

Technique 5: The Leaves on a Stream Exercise

This is a short visualization exercise from mindfulness practice. It takes about two minutes, and it's incredibly helpful for watching thoughts without getting hooked by them.

Sit for a moment and imagine you're sitting beside a gentle stream. Leaves are floating by on the water. Each leaf carries a thought—maybe a worry, maybe a memory, maybe a daydream urge.

Your job is to just watch the leaves float by. Notice each thought. Place it on a leaf. Watch it drift downstream and out of view. Then notice the next thought. Place it on another leaf. Watch it go.

You're not stopping the stream. You're not controlling which thoughts appear. You're just watching them come and go, come and go.

Do this for two minutes. Every time a daydream thought appears, notice it. "There's the thought about the fantasy scene." Place it on a leaf. Let it float away. Don't climb onto the leaf and ride it downstream. Just let it go.

This practice trains you to observe thoughts without engaging. Over time, it gets easier to watch your daydreaming thoughts float by without jumping into them.

Exercise: Titling Your Daydreams

Alright, it's time to get specific about your own fantasy plots. We're going to give them all proper titles, like movies or TV series. This serves two purposes: it helps you recognize patterns, and it creates healthy distance through humor and observation.

Step 1: List Your Recurring Plots

Look back at your Trigger Tracker from Chapter 4. What are the daydream themes that show up repeatedly? Most people have between three and eight main plots that they cycle through.

Write them down. Here are some examples to get you thinking:

- The hero who saves the day
- The romantic relationship where I'm finally understood
- The confrontation where I say exactly the right thing
- The successful professional who impresses everyone
- The creative genius who creates something amazing
- The adventure where I'm brave and capable
- The revenge scenario where the people who hurt me regret it
- The found family where I finally belong

What are yours?

Step 2: Give Each Plot a Movie Title

Now give each plot a title that captures it in a way that's both accurate and slightly humorous. The humor is important—it creates distance and prevents you from taking the plot too seriously.

Examples:

- "Workplace Hero: A Power Fantasy"
- "The Perfect Romance That Could Never Exist"
- "Epic Confrontation, Take 437"
- "Career Triumphs and Total Vindication"
- "Adventure Time: But Make It Escapist"
- "Revenge of the Underestimated"

Be playful with this. The goal isn't to mock yourself. It's to see these plots as stories—fictional narratives your mind keeps offering you—rather than urgent needs you must fulfill.

Step 3: Identify the "Season" or "Episode"

If you've been running the same plots for months or years, you might have different versions or chapters. Name them.

"Oh, this is 'Epic Confrontation,' Season 2, where I've quit the job and they're begging me to come back."

"This is 'Perfect Romance,' the early episodes, before the relationship gets complicated in my fantasy."

Step 4: Use These Titles in Real Time

Once you've named your plots, start using these titles when you notice daydream urges appearing.

"There's 'Workplace Hero' again."

"'Perfect Romance' is trying to pull me in."

"My mind really wants me to watch 'Epic Confrontation' right now."

Every time you use the title, you're practicing defusion. You're observing the story instead of merging with it.

When Defusion Feels Hard

Some days, defusion will be easy. You'll notice the thought, label it, and move on without much effort. Other days, it'll feel nearly impossible. The pull of the fantasy will be so strong that all the defusion techniques in the world won't seem to help.

This is normal.

Defusion isn't about making urges disappear. It's about changing your relationship with them. Some urges are going to be strong because the emotional trigger underneath is strong. If you're feeling intensely lonely, the urge to escape into a fantasy relationship will be powerful. If you're feeling inadequate, the urge to imagine being successful will be compelling.

When the urge is that strong, defusion alone might not be enough. You'll need to combine it with:

1. **An anchoring technique** (from Chapter 5) to ground yourself physically
2. **An understanding of what value you're seeking** (Chapter 7, coming next)
3. **A small action toward that value in real life** (Chapter 8)

All these pieces work together. Defusion creates space between you and the urge. Anchoring brings you into your body. Values clarify what you really need. And committed action starts giving you that thing in reality instead of fantasy.

But defusion is the essential first step. Because if you can't create any space between the urge and your response, the other skills won't have room to work.

The Long Game

You're going to use defusion techniques dozens, maybe hundreds of times over the next few weeks. And initially, it might feel like you're just treading water. The thoughts keep coming. The urges keep appearing. You keep unhooking, and they keep coming back.

Don't lose heart.

What you're doing is retraining your brain. For years, maybe decades, your brain learned: *Daydream thought appears →* *Immediately follow it → Get reward.* That's a strong pattern. You're now building a new pattern: *Daydream thought appears* *→ Notice it → Observe it → Choose not to follow it → Redirect* *to something meaningful.*

New patterns take time to establish. But every single time you practice defusion—every time you notice a thought without acting on it—you're weakening the old pattern and strengthening the new one.

Research on habit change shows that it takes an average of 66 days for a new behavior to become automatic, though this varies widely depending on the complexity of the behavior (Lally et al., 2010). Your brain needs repetition. It needs practice. It needs proof that the new pattern works.

So be patient with yourself. Be consistent with the practice. And trust that the cumulative effect of all these small moments of unhooking will eventually rewire your default response.

You're not trying to stop thoughts from appearing. You're learning to change what you do when they appear.

And that makes all the difference.

What You're Building

Cognitive defusion is the skill of observing your thoughts without automatically acting on them. It creates space between the urge to daydream and your response to that urge—space where choice becomes possible.

Fusion is when you merge with thoughts so completely that you follow them instantly. Defusion is when you see thoughts as mental events—stories your mind offers, not commands you must obey.

The five defusion techniques are: Thank Your Mind, Name the Story, Use "I'm Having the Thought That," Let It Play in the Background, and Leaves on a Stream. Practice all of them and find your favorites.

Give your recurring daydream plots specific titles, like movies. Use these titles in real time when urges appear. This creates distance and helps you observe rather than engage.

Defusion won't make urges disappear, but it changes your relationship with them. You're no longer controlled by every thought your mind generates. You're the one choosing which thoughts deserve action.

Practice defusion consistently, even when it feels hard. You're building a new neural pattern, and that takes time and repetition. Every moment you unhook from a story, you're rewiring your brain.

Now that you can notice the drift, anchor yourself back, and unhook from the stories, we're ready for the most important skill: understanding what your daydreams are really trying to give you. That's next. That's where everything clicks into place.

Chapter 7: Find Your Real-Life "Why" (The "Pivot" Skill 2: Values)

Tom spends his commute home every evening daydreaming about being a war correspondent. In his fantasy, he's brave, decisive, reporting from dangerous places while everyone back home watches in awe. His editor calls him "the best we've got." His colleagues respect him. His family finally understands that he's not just some guy shuffling papers in a cubicle—he's capable of extraordinary things.

In real life, Tom works in data entry at an insurance company. He's never traveled outside his state. He's never written anything more substantial than an email. And he's never told anyone about these fantasies because they seem ridiculous given his actual life.

But here's what Tom doesn't realize: **his daydreams aren't ridiculous. They're a map.**

They're showing him exactly what he's hungry for. And if he can decode that message—if he can figure out what psychological need the fantasy is meeting—he can start building that thing into his real life. Not by becoming a war correspondent (though hey, if that's genuinely what he wants, more power to him), but by finding ways to experience the core feeling that fantasy provides.

This is the chapter where everything changes. This is where you stop fighting your daydreams and start learning from them.

Because **your fantasies are trying to tell you what you value.** They're showing you what's missing from your life. And once you know what you're really seeking, you can start seeking it in ways that actually work.

What Values Actually Are

Before we decode your daydreams, we need to understand what psychologists mean by "values."

Values aren't goals. Goals are things you achieve and then check off your list: "Get promoted. Buy a house. Lose 20 pounds." Values are ongoing directions—ways of living that matter to you, regardless of external outcomes (Harris, 2009).

Think of it this way: **A goal is a destination. A value is a direction you want to keep moving in.**

If your goal is "get married," that's something you either accomplish or don't. But if your value is "connection," that's something you can live into every single day through your actions, regardless of your relationship status. You can experience connection by texting a friend, having a meaningful conversation with a coworker, volunteering with others, or joining a book club. The value isn't something you achieve once and you're done. It's something you express through how you live.

Research in Acceptance and Commitment Therapy identifies values as one of the core components of psychological health (Hayes et al., 2012). People who live in alignment with their values—who regularly take actions that express what matters to them—report higher life satisfaction, better mental health, and greater resilience in the face of stress (Gloster et al., 2017).

People who don't? They feel empty. Disconnected. Like they're going through the motions of life without any real meaning or direction. And guess what they often do to cope with that emptiness?

They escape into fantasy worlds where they *can* experience those values, even if it's only in their imagination.

That's you. That's what's been happening. Your daydreams have been your brain's way of trying to give you what your real life isn't providing.

The Core Human Values

According to Self-Determination Theory, one of the most well-researched frameworks in psychology, humans have three fundamental psychological needs (Ryan & Deci, 2000):

Competence: The need to feel effective, skilled, and capable of mastering challenges **Connection** (or Relatedness): The need for close, meaningful relationships and a sense of belonging **Autonomy**: The need for self-direction, freedom, and control over your own choices

When these needs are met, people thrive. When they're chronically unmet, people suffer—and they often create substitute experiences through fantasy, substance use, excessive gaming, or other forms of escape.

But these three core needs branch out into many specific values that might show up in your life:

- Achievement and mastery
- Creativity and self-expression
- Contribution and making a difference
- Recognition and being seen
- Adventure and novelty
- Justice and fairness
- Growth and learning

- Authenticity and being true to yourself
- Comfort and security
- Fun and pleasure

Your particular daydreams will reflect your particular values. The specific fantasies you create—the roles you play, the scenarios you imagine—are custom-built to meet your specific psychological hungers.

And that's actually beautiful, in a way. Your imagination knows what you need. It's been trying to give it to you. The problem is just that it's been giving you a simulation instead of the real thing.

Decoding Your Daydreams

So how do you figure out which values your daydreams are pointing toward?

You ask a simple question: **"What is this fantasy giving me that my real life isn't?"**

Not on the surface level. Not "it's giving me excitement" or "it's making me feel good." Go deeper. What core human need is being satisfied in this fantasy?

Let's look at some common daydream themes and decode them:

Hero/Savior Fantasies

You daydream about saving people, solving impossible problems, being the one everyone relies on in a crisis. You're competent, skilled, essential.

What value this reveals: Competence, contribution, mattering. You want to feel capable and to know that your abilities make a real difference.

Romance/Relationship Fantasies

You daydream about being in a relationship where you're truly seen and understood. Someone who gets the real you, who appreciates your quirks, who makes you feel less alone.

What value this reveals: Connection, intimacy, belonging. You're hungry for deep relationships where you can be authentic and feel accepted.

Fame/Recognition Fantasies

You daydream about being admired, respected, celebrated for your work or talent. People finally see how special you are. Your worth is undeniable.

What value this reveals: Recognition, validation, significance. You want to be seen and valued for who you are and what you can do.

Confrontation/Revenge Fantasies

You daydream about finally telling someone off, standing up for yourself, or having people who wronged you realize their mistake and apologize.

What value this reveals: Autonomy, justice, self-respect. You want control over your own life and to be treated with the respect you deserve.

Adventure/Escape Fantasies

You daydream about traveling to exotic places, having exciting experiences, living a life full of novelty and stimulation.

What value this reveals: Growth, freedom, vitality. You're craving new experiences and the feeling of being fully alive.

Creative/Artistic Success Fantasies

You daydream about creating something amazing—a novel, a painting, a business—that shows the world your unique vision and talent.

What value this reveals: Creativity, self-expression, legacy. You want to create something meaningful that reflects who you are.

Power/Control Fantasies

You daydream about being in charge, making important decisions, having authority and resources to shape outcomes.

What value this reveals: Autonomy, impact, self-direction. You want agency in your own life and the ability to influence your circumstances.

See the pattern? **Every fantasy is trying to meet a legitimate psychological need.** The fantasies themselves might be unrealistic or impossible, but the underlying needs are completely valid. You're not broken for wanting these things. You're human.

The problem is just that you've been trying to satisfy these needs in a way that doesn't actually work. Simulated competence doesn't make you feel competent in real life. Imaginary connection doesn't ease loneliness. Fantasy recognition doesn't build genuine self-esteem.

You need the real thing.

The Daydream Decoder Exercise

Alright, time to get specific about your own fantasies. We're going to translate your recurring daydream plots into the values they represent.

Pull out the list of daydream plots you titled back in Chapter 6. Now we're going to decode what each one is really about.

Step 1: List Your Main Fantasy Themes

Write down your 3-5 most frequent daydream plots. Use the titles you created, or just describe them briefly.

Example:

1. "The Workplace Hero" - I solve a major problem and everyone recognizes how valuable I am
2. "The Perfect Romance" - I'm in a relationship where I'm completely understood and loved
3. "The Great Escape" - I travel the world, free from all my current responsibilities

Step 2: Ask the Decoding Question

For each fantasy, ask: "What is this giving me that my real life isn't?"

Be honest. Go deep. What feeling, what experience, what need is being satisfied here?

Example:

1. "The Workplace Hero" → This is giving me a sense of competence and recognition. In real life, I feel invisible at work and like my contributions don't matter.
2. "The Perfect Romance" → This is giving me connection and acceptance. In real life, I feel lonely and like no one really knows the real me.

3. "The Great Escape" → This is giving me freedom and adventure. In real life, I feel trapped by obligations and routine.

Step 3: Name the Value

Based on what the fantasy is giving you, identify the core value it represents. Use the list from earlier in this chapter, or come up with your own words.

Example:

1. "The Workplace Hero" → **Values: Competence, Recognition, Contribution**
2. "The Perfect Romance" → **Values: Connection, Intimacy, Acceptance**
3. "The Great Escape" → **Values: Freedom, Adventure, Growth**

Do this for all your main fantasies. What you'll probably discover is that you have 2-4 core values that show up repeatedly across different fantasies. These are your big ones—the needs that, when unmet, drive you to escape into fantasy.

Step 4: Get Specific About the Feeling

For each value, describe what experiencing that value would actually feel like in real life. Not what it would look like externally, but how you would feel internally.

Example:

- **Competence**: I would feel confident, capable, like I can handle challenges. I'd trust myself.
- **Connection**: I would feel understood, less alone, like I have people who really get me.

- **Freedom**: I would feel light, unencumbered, like I have choices and aren't trapped.

This matters because when we start building real-world actions (next chapter), we're going to aim for actions that create these feelings, not necessarily the exact scenarios from your fantasies.

When Your Values Conflict with Reality

Sometimes people decode their fantasies and discover values that feel impossible to fulfill given their current circumstances.

"My value is adventure and freedom, but I have three kids and a mortgage. I can't just quit everything and travel the world."

"My value is creative self-expression, but I work 60 hours a week at a job that has nothing to do with creativity. There's no time."

"My value is connection, but I have social anxiety and making friends is terrifying."

Here's what you need to understand: **Values aren't about dramatic life overhauls. They're about small, consistent actions in the direction that matters to you.**

You don't have to quit your job and move to Bali to honor a value of freedom. You can make small choices each day that increase your sense of autonomy and agency. You can say no to one obligation you've been taking on out of guilt. You can schedule one afternoon a month to do exactly what you want. You can make a decision about your own life without asking permission.

You don't have to become a famous artist to honor a value of creativity. You can set aside 15 minutes before work to sketch or write. You can approach a problem at your job with creative thinking. You can rearrange your living room in a way that expresses your aesthetic.

You don't have to have a huge friend group to honor a value of connection. You can have one meaningful conversation with one person. You can send a text to someone you've been thinking about. You can show up authentically in one interaction instead of hiding behind a mask.

Values are directions, not destinations. You move toward them through small actions, over and over, in whatever way your current life allows. And over time, those small actions add up to a life that feels meaningful—a life that doesn't need escaping from.

The Most Important Thing You Need to Know

Your values aren't your fantasy scenarios. This is crucial.

Your value isn't "being a famous rock star." Your value is probably recognition, or self-expression, or connection with an audience, or mastery of a craft. The rock star fantasy is just one imaginary way to experience those values.

Which means you can experience those same values in many other ways—ways that are actually accessible to you in real life.

Claire daydreamed constantly about being a bestselling author with millions of readers. When she decoded this, she realized her values were creative self-expression and making an impact on people's lives. She didn't actually need millions of readers. She needed to create something meaningful and share it with others.

So she started a blog. Ten people read it regularly. Then twenty. It wasn't millions, but it was real. She was expressing herself creatively and getting genuine feedback from actual humans who connected with her words. The need was being met in reality, not fantasy. And the pull of the daydream weakened.

David daydreamed about being a CEO, making big decisions, commanding respect. His values were autonomy and impact. He didn't need to be a CEO. He needed more agency in his life and a sense that his actions mattered.

So he started small. He took on a leadership role in a volunteer organization. He made decisions about his own schedule instead of defaulting to what others wanted. He spoke up in meetings at work instead of staying silent. Tiny acts of autonomy and impact. The fantasy lost its urgency.

The fantasy is a costume the value wears. You don't need the costume. You need the value.

And the beautiful thing about values is that they're infinitely flexible. There are a thousand ways to experience competence, connection, freedom, creativity. You're not locked into one specific path. You just need to start taking actions—any actions—that move you in the direction of what matters.

What If You Don't Know Your Values?

Some people go through this exercise and draw a blank. They can't figure out what their fantasies are really about. Or they identify a value but it doesn't feel quite right.

That's okay. Values clarification isn't always immediate. Sometimes you need to experiment.

Here are some additional questions that might help:

- **When have you felt most alive and engaged in your real life?** What were you doing? What values might that reflect?

- **What makes you angry or sad about the world?**
  Often, what upsets us points to what we care about. If
  injustice makes you angry, justice might be a value. If
  loneliness makes you sad, connection might be a value.
- **If you had one year to live and you knew you couldn't
  fail at anything you tried, what would you do?** Not for
  external reasons—not for money or fame—but because it
  mattered to you. What does that tell you about your
  values?
- **Whose life do you envy, and why?** Not the surface stuff
  (their house, their appearance), but the way they spend
  their time, what they prioritize, how they show up in the
  world. What value might that envy be pointing toward?

You can also just pick a value and test it. "Maybe my value is
growth and learning. Let me try taking one action this week
toward learning something new and see how it feels." If it feels
meaningful and satisfying, you're probably on the right track. If
it feels empty or forced, try a different value.

Values aren't something you figure out once and you're done.
They can shift over time as you change and grow. The important
thing is to start somewhere and pay attention to what resonates.

The Shift That's Happening

If you do this exercise honestly—if you really decode what your
fantasies are trying to give you—something shifts.

You stop seeing your daydreams as random, shameful escapism.
You start seeing them as messengers. They're showing you what
you're hungry for. They're pointing toward what your life needs
more of.

And that changes the whole game.

Instead of beating yourself up for daydreaming, you can get curious: "Huh, I'm really pulled toward that hero fantasy today. What does that tell me? Maybe I'm feeling incompetent about something. Maybe I need to do something that makes me feel capable."

Instead of feeling stuck in your fantasies, you can ask: "What does this fantasy give me, and how can I get a taste of that in real life today?"

Your fantasies stop being the problem and start being the solution. They're diagnostic tools. They tell you what you're missing. And once you know what you're missing, you can start building it.

That's the Pivot. That's how you make your real life more compelling than your fantasy. Not by forcing yourself to be grateful for a life that isn't meeting your needs, but by actively reshaping your life to include more of what matters to you.

Small actions. Consistent direction. Real experiences of the values your fantasies have been simulating.

In the next chapter, we'll turn these values into concrete actions you can take today. But for now, just sit with what you've discovered. Look at your values. Feel the truth of them.

These aren't just words on a page. These are the things that make life worth living for you. These are what you've been seeking all along.

Now you know what you're looking for. And that changes everything.

What You've Discovered

Your daydreams aren't random or meaningless—they're showing you what you value. They're trying to give you experiences that your real life isn't providing. Every fantasy reflects an unmet psychological need.

Values are directions, not destinations. They're ongoing ways of living that matter to you. The three fundamental human needs are competence, connection, and autonomy, but these branch into many specific values like creativity, recognition, adventure, justice, and growth.

To decode your daydreams, ask: "What is this fantasy giving me that my real life isn't?" Then identify the core value that fantasy represents. Your recurring fantasies probably point to 2-4 core values that are currently unmet in your life.

The fantasy scenario (being a rock star, being a hero, having a perfect romance) is just the costume. The value underneath is what you really need. And values can be experienced in countless ways that are actually accessible to you.

Values aren't about dramatic life changes. They're about small, consistent actions that move you in the direction that matters. You don't need to become your fantasy to experience your values. You just need to take real steps toward what you care about.

Your daydreams are messengers, not enemies. They're diagnostic tools showing you what your life needs more of. Now that you know your values, you can start building them into reality.

In the next chapter, we'll translate these values into specific, tiny actions you can take today to start experiencing what matters to you in real life instead of fantasy.

Chapter 8: Build a Better "Real" (The "Pivot" Skill 3: Committed Action)

You know your values now. You've decoded what your daydreams are really trying to give you. You understand what you're hungry for.

So what now?

This is where most people get stuck. They think: "Okay, my value is connection, but I'm lonely and I don't have close friends, so... now what? Do I completely rebuild my social life? How do I even start? This is overwhelming."

Or: "My value is competence, but I'm stuck in a job where I feel useless. Do I quit? Go back to school? Learn a new skill? I don't have time or money for major changes."

And because the gap between "my life as it is" and "my life as I wish it were" feels impossibly huge, they do nothing. Or they try to make a massive change all at once, burn out after a week, and slip right back into daydreaming.

Here's what you need to understand: You're not trying to close the gap overnight. You're trying to take one step—one tiny, doable step—in the direction of your values today.

That's it. Not tomorrow's step. Not next month's step. Just today's step.

Because here's the thing about values: you don't achieve them. You live them through your actions, moment by moment, day by day. And even the smallest action in the direction of what matters is enough to start weakening the pull of fantasy.

This is called *committed action* in ACT, and it's the final piece of the Pivot (Wilson & DuFrene, 2009). You're not building a perfect life. You're building a life that's good enough, meaningful enough, fulfilling enough that you don't need to escape from it constantly.

Why Tiny Actions Matter

Let's talk about why small actions work when big intentions don't.

Your brain operates on a reward-based learning system. It does things that produce good feelings and avoids things that produce bad feelings (Schultz, 2015). Right now, your brain has learned that daydreaming produces fast, reliable rewards—relief from discomfort plus a hit of fulfillment. Real life, by comparison, has been producing slow, uncertain, often disappointing results.

So your brain keeps choosing fantasy. It's the logical choice given the data.

To change this, you need to give your brain new data. You need to show it that real life can also produce good feelings—maybe not as intense or immediate as fantasy, but real, genuine, lasting satisfaction.

But here's the trick: **the action has to be small enough that you'll actually do it.**

If you set a goal like "make three new close friends this month," your brain looks at that and thinks, "That's terrifying, time-consuming, and likely to result in rejection and failure. Hard pass. Let's daydream instead."

But if you set a goal like "send one text to someone I used to be friendly with," your brain thinks, "Okay, that's five minutes and not particularly risky. I can do that."

And when you do it—when you send that text and maybe get a friendly response back—you get a small hit of real connection. Your brain notes: "Huh. Real action produced real reward. Interesting."

One data point. That's all. But it's a start.

Do it again tomorrow. Another small action. Another real reward. More data.

Over time, your brain starts to recalibrate. Real life becomes more rewarding. The gap between fantasy rewards and reality rewards shrinks. And the compulsive pull toward daydreaming weakens, not because you're fighting it harder, but because you're getting what you need from reality now.

This is supported by research on behavioral activation, which shows that engaging in small, values-based activities—even when you don't feel like it—reduces depression, anxiety, and avoidance behaviors (Lejuez et al., 2011). Action creates motivation, not the other way around. You don't wait until you feel motivated to act. You act, and motivation follows.

The 5-Minute Rule

Here's your guideline for committed actions: **Can I do this in five minutes or less?**

If yes, it's the right size. If no, make it smaller.

Five minutes is short enough that you can't procrastinate it into oblivion. You can't say "I don't have time" because everyone has five minutes. And it's short enough that even if it doesn't go perfectly, you haven't lost much.

But five minutes is also long enough to do something real. You can send a text, do a quick sketch, listen to one song mindfully, read two pages of a book, practice one skill, make one decision about your own life.

These actions might seem laughably small compared to the grand fantasies you've been living in. You've been imagining yourself as a bestselling author, and now you're supposed to be satisfied with writing for five minutes?

Yes. Exactly yes.

Because **the feeling you get from five minutes of real action is more nourishing than five hours of fantasy.** The fantasy gives you a simulation of accomplishment. The real action gives you actual accomplishment. Your brain knows the difference, even if you don't consciously realize it.

And here's the thing: small actions have a way of building momentum. You write for five minutes and it feels good, so tomorrow you write for seven minutes. Then ten. Then you're writing regularly, and six months later you've actually finished something real. Not a fantasy novel you've been imagining for years—an actual draft of actual words.

Small actions compound. They add up. They create confidence. "I said I'd do something and I did it. I'm someone who follows through." That identity shift is powerful.

Turning Values into Actions

Let's take each common value and break it down into tiny, specific actions you can take today.

If Your Value Is Connection:

- Send one text to someone you've been thinking about. Just "Hey, thinking of you. Hope you're well."
- Have one real conversation with someone instead of staying surface-level. Ask one genuine question and actually listen to the answer.
- Make eye contact and smile at someone you pass today. Real human acknowledgment.
- Join one online community related to something you care about and make one comment.
- Call a family member you haven't talked to in a while, even for just five minutes.

If Your Value Is Competence:

- Practice one skill for five minutes. Doesn't matter which skill. Just practice.
- Complete one small task you've been avoiding. Cross it off your list and notice how that feels.
- Ask one question about something you don't understand. Seeking to learn is an act of competence.
- Help someone with something you're good at. Teaching reinforces mastery.
- Try one thing you're not sure you can do. Even if you fail, you'll learn.

If Your Value Is Creativity:

- Create something for five minutes. Draw, write, make music, take a photo, rearrange a space. Anything.
- Engage with someone else's creative work and really pay attention to it. Read a poem slowly. Look at a painting. Listen to an album.
- Solve one problem in a novel way. Approach a routine task differently.

- Write down one idea, even if it seems silly. Ideas are creative sparks.
- Experiment with something. Try a new recipe, a new route to work, a new way of doing something familiar.

If Your Value Is Autonomy:

- Make one decision today that's entirely yours, without asking permission or seeking approval.
- Say no to one thing you don't actually want to do.
- Choose something about your environment. Move furniture, change your desktop wallpaper, wear something you like.
- Spend five minutes doing exactly what you want, with no agenda or productivity goal.
- Set one boundary with someone. "I'm not available for that" or "I need some space right now."

If Your Value Is Recognition:

- Share one thing you've done with someone. Show them your work, tell them about an accomplishment, let yourself be seen.
- Give yourself one genuine compliment out loud. Recognize yourself even if no one else does.
- Ask for feedback on something. This is an act of self-respect—believing your work is worth others' attention.
- Celebrate one small win today, even if it's tiny. Notice it. Mark it.
- Post something you created or an achievement on social media. (Or don't. But if you want recognition, sometimes you have to make yourself visible.)

If Your Value Is Growth:

- Learn one new thing today. Watch a tutorial, read an article, ask someone to explain something.

- Try something uncomfortable. Step slightly outside your comfort zone in any area.
- Reflect for five minutes on what you learned from a recent experience.
- Read two pages of a book in an area you want to grow in.
- Sign up for one thing—a class, a workshop, a webinar, a challenge. Commit to showing up.

If Your Value Is Adventure:

- Do one thing differently today. Take a different route, try a new food, change your routine.
- Research one place you'd like to visit. Even if you can't go now, the planning is part of the adventure.
- Say yes to one invitation or opportunity you'd normally decline.
- Explore one small thing in your area you've never checked out. A park, a coffee shop, a street.
- Break one small rule that doesn't actually matter. (Not a law. Just a personal pattern you've been rigidly following.)

See how these work? They're specific, concrete, and doable today. You're not overhauling your life. You're taking one action that expresses what matters to you.

The Pivot Plan Worksheet

Time to build your personal action plan. This is where theory becomes practice.

Step 1: Choose Your Top Value

From the work you did in Chapter 7, pick the value that feels most urgent right now. Which one, if you started experiencing it more in real life, would most reduce your need to escape into fantasy?

Write it down: **My current priority value is:** _____

Step 2: Identify Three 5-Minute Actions

Come up with three specific actions you could take this week that would move you toward this value. Each one should take five minutes or less.

Make them concrete. Not "be more social" but "text Emma and ask how she's doing." Not "be creative" but "write one paragraph of the story idea I've been thinking about."

Example (if your value is Connection):

1. Text Jordan and ask if he wants to grab coffee sometime
2. Have a real conversation with one coworker instead of small talk
3. Call Mom on Wednesday evening

Step 3: Schedule Them

This is crucial. Don't just write down the actions and hope you'll do them. Put them in your calendar. Decide exactly when.

Monday 7pm: Text Jordan Wednesday lunch: Real conversation with coworker Wednesday 8pm: Call Mom

Research on implementation intentions shows that people who specify when and where they'll do something are much more likely to follow through (Gollwitzer & Sheeran, 2006). "I will do X at Y time in Z place" is far more effective than "I should do X sometime."

Step 4: Track What Happens

After each action, write down:

- Did you do it? (Yes/No)
- How did it feel? (What emotions came up?)
- Did it satisfy the value even a little bit? (Did you feel a hint of connection, competence, etc.?)

You're gathering data again. You're showing your brain that real action produces real results.

Step 5: Adjust and Repeat

At the end of the week, look at your data. What worked? What didn't? Do you need to make the actions smaller? Try different ones? Focus on a different value?

Then plan the next week. Three more actions. Schedule them. Do them. Track them.

This becomes your rhythm. Week after week. Small actions, consistent direction, building a life that reflects what matters to you.

When Actions Feel Empty

Sometimes you'll take an action and it won't feel satisfying. You'll text someone and they won't respond. You'll try something new and it'll be disappointing. You'll practice a skill and feel more incompetent than before you started.

This is normal. Not every action produces an immediate good feeling. Real life is messy and unpredictable. That's actually one of the reasons fantasy has been so appealing—it's reliable.

But here's what you need to keep in mind: **Values aren't about outcomes. They're about direction.**

You can't control whether someone texts you back. But you can control whether you reach out. Reaching out is the value-aligned action. That's what counts.

You can't control whether you're immediately good at a new skill. But you can control whether you practice. The practice itself is the expression of your value, regardless of the result.

When an action doesn't produce the outcome you wanted, you have two choices:

1. **Try again with a different action.** Maybe texting Jordan didn't work, but what about texting Alex? Or showing up to that meetup group?
2. **Trust that consistency matters more than any single instance.** You're building patterns, not chasing perfect moments. Ten actions that feel "meh" are still more valuable than zero actions.

And here's something surprising: even actions that feel empty are still weakening the pull of fantasy. You're proving to yourself that you can engage with reality instead of escaping it. You're practicing showing up. That has value even when it's not immediately rewarding.

The Gap Between Fantasy and Reality

Your daydreams are incredibly satisfying. They're perfectly tailored to give you exactly what you want, exactly when you want it. Real life will never feel that smooth or that perfectly satisfying.

And that's okay.

You're not trying to make real life feel as good as fantasy. You're trying to make it good enough that you don't need the fantasy as desperately.

103

It's like the difference between eating real food versus looking at pictures of food when you're starving. The pictures might look more perfect—idealized, Instagram-filtered, glossy—but they don't feed you. Real food might be messier, less photogenic, but it actually nourishes you.

That's what these small actions are. They're real nourishment. They're not as intense or perfect as the fantasy, but they're actually feeding the needs your daydreams have been simulating.

Over time, as you consistently take values-based actions, the fantasy's appeal fades. Not because you're fighting it harder, but because you're less hungry. You're getting fed in reality.

And the amazing thing is, once you're less dependent on the fantasy for psychological survival, you can actually enjoy it differently. (We'll talk about this more in Chapter 9.) You can use your imagination for creative projects, for problem-solving, for brief mental breaks—all on purpose, all in ways you control.

But first, you have to start feeding yourself in reality. Small actions. This week. Today.

What You're Building

Committed action means taking small, specific steps in the direction of your values. You're not trying to achieve perfection or close the gap between your life and your ideal all at once. You're just taking the next right step, over and over.

Small actions work because they're doable, they produce real (not simulated) rewards, and they give your brain new data: real life can be satisfying too. Use the 5-minute rule—if it takes longer than five minutes, make it smaller.

Every value can be expressed through tiny actions today. Connection, competence, creativity, autonomy, recognition, growth, adventure—all of these can be experienced in small, accessible ways.

Create your Pivot Plan: choose your top value, identify three 5-minute actions for this week, schedule them, do them, track what happens, and adjust as needed. Repeat weekly.

Not every action will feel immediately satisfying. That's okay. Values are about direction, not outcomes. Consistency matters more than perfection. You're building patterns and proving to yourself that you can show up in reality.

Real life will never feel as perfectly satisfying as fantasy, and that's fine. You're not trying to match the fantasy. You're trying to make reality good enough that you don't desperately need the escape anymore.

In the next chapter, we'll talk about how to harness your creative imagination for productive purposes instead of letting it run wild. Your creativity isn't the enemy—it's a resource. Let's learn how to use it.

Chapter 9: Harness Your Creative Fire

We need to talk about what happens to your imagination after you've learned to anchor yourself, unhook from stories, identify your values, and take committed action.

Because here's the thing: **your imagination isn't going away.** Nor should it.

That vivid, powerful, creative capacity you have? That's not a bug. That's not the problem. The problem has been that this incredible resource has been running on autopilot, using you instead of you using it.

But what if you could redirect it? What if you could take that same imaginative energy and channel it into something genuinely creative—something that leaves you with actual output, actual accomplishment, actual contribution to the world?

That's what this chapter is about. We're not killing your daydreaming. We're teaching you how to schedule it, contain it, and transform it from compulsive escape into intentional creation.

The Creativity Hidden in Your Daydreams

You've been creating elaborate narratives in your head for months, maybe years, maybe decades. Complex characters. Intricate plots. Emotional depth. Rich sensory detail. That's not nothing. **That's the work of a creative mind.**

Research shows that people with maladaptive daydreaming often score high on measures of creativity, fantasy-proneness, and imaginative absorption (Bigelsen et al., 2016). You're not daydreaming because you're uncreative. You're daydreaming partly *because* you're highly creative and your mind is constantly generating rich inner content.

The question is: what are you doing with that creativity?

Right now, you're letting it evaporate. You create these amazing scenes and stories and then... nothing. They disappear. You get nothing tangible from the hours you spend imagining. It's like cooking elaborate meals every day and then throwing them in the trash before you eat them. All that effort, all that creativity, and nothing to show for it.

But what if you captured it? What if you took those storylines and wrote them down? Painted them? Turned them into something concrete that exists outside your head?

This isn't just about productivity. This is about honoring the creative gift you actually have. Your imagination has been trying to tell you something: *you're meant to create things*. You've just been creating them in the wrong medium—in fantasy instead of reality.

The Difference Between Compulsive and Intentional Daydreaming

Let's be clear about what we're doing here. We're drawing a line between two very different activities:

Compulsive daydreaming:

- Happens automatically in response to triggers
- Lasts as long as it wants, eating up hours
- Leaves you with nothing tangible

- Makes you feel guilty and out of control afterward
- Interferes with responsibilities and relationships
- Is driven by the need to escape discomfort

Intentional creative imagination:

- Happens when you decide it happens
- Has set boundaries (time limits, specific purpose)
- Produces something real (writing, art, problem-solving)
- Makes you feel satisfied and accomplished afterward
- Fits into your life without disrupting it
- Is driven by the desire to create or solve problems

Same basic mental capacity. Totally different relationship to it.

Right now, your daydreaming is like a river that's flooding its banks, destroying everything in its path. What we're going to do is build a channel—a defined path where that creative energy can flow productively without overwhelming your life.

The Container & Channel Method

This is a simple but powerful technique for transforming compulsive daydreaming into productive creativity. It has two parts: the Container (boundaries) and the Channel (productive outlet).

Part 1: The Container

You're going to schedule specific time for daydreaming. Yes, schedule it. Put it on your calendar.

"But won't that just encourage it?"

No. Right now, your daydreaming is uncontrolled and unlimited. Any time, any trigger, for as long as it wants. By scheduling it, you're creating boundaries. You're saying: "This is when daydreaming happens. Not constantly. Not whenever. During this scheduled time."

Start with 30 minutes, three times a week. (You can adjust based on what works for you, but start here.)

Tuesday 7pm: Creative time
Thursday 7pm: Creative time
Saturday 10am: Creative time

These are your designated times for letting your imagination run. Outside these times, when you notice the urge to drift, you can remind yourself: "Not now. I have creative time scheduled for Thursday. I'll explore this then."

This actually makes it easier to resist compulsive drifts. Your mind isn't being told "never." It's being told "not now, but yes later." That's much easier to accept.

Part 2: The Channel

During your scheduled creative time, you're not just going to lie there and daydream. You're going to channel that imaginative energy into something concrete.

Here are your options:

Option 1: Write It Down

Set a timer for 30 minutes. Open a document. Write down the daydream as if you're writing a story. Describe the scene, the dialogue, what the characters are thinking and feeling.

Don't worry about it being good. Don't worry about anyone ever reading it. Just get it out of your head and onto the page.

What this does: It satisfies the creative urge while producing something tangible. You're still engaging with your fantasy world, but now you have a document at the end. That's real. That counts.

And here's what people often discover: **writing it down makes it less compulsive.** Once it's captured on the page, your mind stops obsessively returning to it. It's like your brain was afraid of losing the story, so it kept replaying it. Once it's documented, that anxiety fades.

Option 2: Draw or Sketch It

If you're visual, spend your creative time sketching scenes from your daydreams. The characters, the settings, key moments. Even stick figures are fine.

Again, this captures the imaginary content in a concrete form. You're creating, not just consuming your own mental movies.

Option 3: Use It for Actual Creative Projects

Maybe you've always wanted to write a novel, make a comic, compose music, create a game. Your daydream content could be raw material for that.

Spend your scheduled creative time actually working on the project. Use the characters and scenarios from your daydreams as inspiration, but shape them into something you can share with the world.

This is where the magic happens. You're taking the same creative energy and redirecting it into something productive and potentially fulfilling.

Option 4: Problem-Solving Mode

If your daydreams aren't narrative-driven but more about ideal scenarios (the perfect career, the dream relationship, the life you wish you had), use your creative time to problem-solve.

Set the timer. Grab a notebook. Write: "If I could create my ideal [career/relationship/life], what would it look like? What steps could I take in reality to move closer to that vision?"

You're using your imagination deliberately to generate ideas and solutions, not to escape.

The Power of Time Limits

The timer is not optional. This is crucial.

When you daydream without limits, it's easy to lose three, four, five hours. Time evaporates. But when you set a 30-minute timer, something interesting happens: **your mind actually becomes more focused and productive.**

Research on time constraints shows that they often enhance creativity rather than hinder it (Amabile et al., 2002). When you have unlimited time, you meander. When you have a defined window, you make the most of it.

Plus, knowing the creative time will end makes it easier to engage fully. "It's only 30 minutes" removes the guilt. You're not abandoning your responsibilities for hours. You're taking a brief, scheduled creative break.

And when the timer goes off, you stop. Even if you're in the middle of something. Especially if you're in the middle of something. This trains your brain that you're in control of the creative time, not the other way around.

At first, stopping might feel impossible. "But I'm just getting into it!" Your mind will beg for more time. Don't give in. Stop at

111

30 minutes. Close the document. Stand up. Move on to your next activity.

This is the boundary. This is you being in charge.

Over time, it gets easier. Your mind learns that creative time has limits. And paradoxically, this makes the time you do have more satisfying and productive.

When You Feel Resistance

You might feel resistance to scheduling creative time. Common thoughts:

"This feels silly. I'm an adult. I shouldn't need to schedule daydreaming."

"I don't want to write it down. That's not the same as experiencing it."

"What if 30 minutes isn't enough? What if I get more obsessed?"

"I don't have time for this."

Let's address these:

"This feels silly." Lots of effective things feel silly at first. The question isn't whether it feels silly. The question is whether it works. Try it for two weeks and see.

"Writing it down isn't the same." Correct. It's not the same. That's the point. You're learning to engage with your creative content differently—not as a mental escape, but as raw material for something real.

"What if 30 minutes isn't enough?" Then you'll be uncomfortable when the timer goes off. Good. That discomfort

112

is you learning to tolerate delayed gratification. The urge will pass. And you'll have another scheduled session in a few days.

"I don't have time." You're spending hours a day daydreaming unintentionally. You're replacing that with 30 minutes of intentional creative time. You're not adding to your schedule. You're redirecting what's already happening.

Additional Creative Outlets

Beyond the Container & Channel method, there are other ways to redirect your imaginative energy:

Creative Hobbies:

- Writing (fiction, poetry, blogging)
- Visual art (drawing, painting, digital art)
- Music (composing, learning an instrument)
- Crafting (knitting, woodworking, building things)
- Performance (theater, storytelling, stand-up comedy)

Problem-Solving Activities:

- Strategy games that require creative thinking
- Puzzles and escape rooms
- Brainstorming solutions for real challenges in your life or work
- Learning skills that require creativity (cooking, design, coding)

Structured Imagination:

- Role-playing games (D&D and similar games let you use your imagination collaboratively and with structure)
- Improvisational activities
- Writing prompts or creative challenges

The key is that these activities give your creativity a productive outlet with boundaries and real output. You're using your imaginative capacity, but you're directing it toward something tangible.

The Shift from Escape to Expression

As you practice scheduled creative time and redirect your imagination into productive channels, something shifts in how you relate to your creativity.

It stops being a shameful escape and starts being a genuine gift. You stop hiding your imaginative capacity and start expressing it. You stop feeling controlled by your fantasies and start using them as fuel for actual creative work.

And here's what's beautiful: **the more you channel your creativity into real projects, the less you need the compulsive daydreaming.**

Why? Because you're getting something real from your imagination now. You're building a body of work. You're developing skills. You might even be sharing your creations with others and getting real feedback, real recognition, real connection.

The fantasy world loses its desperate appeal when you're creating things in the real world that actually satisfy your creative hunger.

This is the full transformation. You went from being controlled by MD to being in charge of your imagination. You went from escaping reality to enriching reality with your creativity.

Your imagination isn't the enemy. It never was. It's a powerful resource that needed better direction. Now you're giving it that direction.

Moving Forward with Your Creative Power

Your imagination is a genuine creative gift. People with MD often score high on creativity measures. The problem hasn't been that you're too creative—it's that your creativity has been channeled into compulsive escape instead of productive expression.

The Container & Channel method gives your imagination boundaries and direction. Schedule 30-minute creative sessions 2-3 times per week. During those times, channel your daydreams into something concrete: writing, art, problem-solving, or creative projects.

The timer is essential. Work for exactly 30 minutes, then stop. This trains your brain that you're in control of creative time, not the other way around. Time limits actually enhance creativity and focus.

There's a difference between compulsive daydreaming (automatic, endless, guilt-inducing) and intentional creative imagination (scheduled, bounded, productive). Same mental capacity, totally different relationship to it.

The more you channel creativity into real projects with real output, the less you'll need compulsive daydreaming. You're getting genuine satisfaction from creating things in reality that actually feed your creative hunger.

Your imagination isn't the enemy. It's a resource. Now you know how to use it.

In the next chapter, we'll talk about what happens when you slip—when you lose a day to daydreaming despite all these tools. Because you will. Everyone does. And knowing how to recover with compassion instead of shame is essential.

Chapter 10: The Relapse & Recovery Plan

It's going to happen. You know it's going to happen. So let's plan for it now.

You're going to have a day—maybe many days—where you lose hours to daydreaming despite everything you've learned. You'll use all the tools. You'll notice the drift, try to anchor, attempt to unhook from the story. And it won't work. The pull will be too strong. You'll give in. And you'll lose the afternoon, the evening, maybe the whole day to fantasy.

Then the shame will hit. The familiar crushing disappointment in yourself. "I learned all these techniques and I still can't stop. I'm hopeless. This is never going to change. I might as well give up."

Stop right there.

That shame spiral? That's the real problem. Not the relapse itself. The relapse is normal, predictable, part of the process. The shame is what keeps you stuck.

So we're going to build a relapse and recovery plan now, before it happens, so you know exactly what to do when you drift. This plan has four steps, and it's designed to get you back on track quickly without the usual self-destruction.

Step 1: Notice (Without the Drama)

First, you need to notice that you've drifted. Sometimes this happens in real-time—you catch yourself mid-daydream.

Sometimes it happens after the fact—you "wake up" and realize several hours have passed.

Either way, your job is to notice without adding a dramatic story on top of it.

What your mind will want to say:
"Oh my god, I did it again. I'm such a failure. I knew this wouldn't work. I'll always be like this. I'm broken. There's no point even trying. I might as well just—"

What you're going to say instead:
"I drifted. That happened. Okay."

That's it. Just the facts. No interpretation. No catastrophizing. No character assassination. You drifted. Period.

This is called *self-compassion*, and research shows it's one of the most powerful predictors of sustained behavior change (Neff & Germer, 2013). People who respond to setbacks with self-compassion rather than self-criticism are more likely to get back on track quickly and maintain progress long-term.

Think about how you'd respond if a good friend told you they relapsed into an old pattern. Would you say, "You're hopeless and pathetic"? Or would you say, "That's tough. It happens. What do you think triggered it?"

Treat yourself the way you'd treat that friend. With kindness. With curiosity. Without drama.

Helpful phrases for this stage:

- "I'm human. Humans have setbacks."
- "One day doesn't erase all my progress."
- "I can learn from this and do better tomorrow."
- "This is part of the process, not proof of failure."

Step 2: Anchor (Get Back in Your Body)

Once you've noticed the drift without spiraling into shame, the next step is to ground yourself physically. Remember the anchoring techniques from Chapter 5? Use one now.

This serves two purposes:

Purpose 1: It interrupts the drift. Even if you've been daydreaming for hours, you can still anchor yourself in the present moment right now. Feel your feet on the floor. Do the 5-4-3-2-1 sensory check. Run cold water on your hands. Get back into your body.

Purpose 2: It proves you're capable of redirecting. The shame voice wants you to believe you're powerless. By anchoring, you prove that's not true. You can redirect your attention. You just did. That's a win, even on a bad day.

Don't skip this step. Even if you feel like it's too late, that the day is already ruined, anchor yourself anyway. You're practicing the skill. You're proving to yourself that you're not completely at the mercy of your mind.

Plus, anchoring helps reduce the emotional intensity that often follows a relapse. When you're overwhelmed with shame and frustration, your body is flooded with stress hormones. Anchoring techniques activate your parasympathetic nervous system, which calms you down (Porges, 2011). You literally can't problem-solve or plan next steps effectively when you're in fight-or-flight mode. Anchor first, then think.

Step 3: Get Curious About the Value You Were Missing

Here's where it gets interesting. Instead of beating yourself up, you're going to investigate.

Ask yourself: **"What was I feeling right before I drifted? What value was I seeking?"**

Every relapse has a trigger. Always. You didn't just randomly start daydreaming. Something was happening—externally or internally—that created a need to escape.

Maybe you were stressed about a work deadline (seeking relief from discomfort).
Maybe you were lonely on a Friday night (seeking connection).
Maybe you felt inadequate after comparing yourself to someone (seeking competence or recognition).
Maybe you were just bored and understimulated (seeking novelty or meaning).

Whatever it was, **your daydream was trying to meet a real need.** It just met it in a way that doesn't actually work long-term.

Get curious about what that need was. Don't judge it. Don't dismiss it. Just notice: "Oh, I was feeling X, and my brain automatically reached for the daydream as a way to cope with X."

This transforms the relapse from a failure into information. You're gathering data about what triggers you, what you need, and where your weak spots are.

Write it down if that helps:

"Today I drifted for 3 hours. Right before I drifted, I was feeling _____. The value I was seeking was _____. My brain tried to give me that through daydreaming about _____."

This is not about making excuses. This is about understanding patterns so you can interrupt them next time.

Step 4: Make a New Pivot Plan

Now that you know what value was missing, you can make a plan for how to meet that need in reality instead of fantasy.

This is where you return to the Pivot Plan from Chapter 8. You're going to identify one small action you can take today— right now, if possible—that moves you toward the value you were seeking.

Example:

"I drifted because I was feeling lonely. My value is connection. Right now, I'm going to text Maria and ask if she wants to meet for coffee this weekend."

"I drifted because I was feeling incompetent at work. My value is competence. Right now, I'm going to complete one small task on my to-do list to prove I can accomplish something."

"I drifted because I was bored and understimulated. My value is growth/novelty. Right now, I'm going to spend 10 minutes learning something new—maybe watch a tutorial or read an article about something I'm curious about."

The action needs to be small and immediate. Not "I'll fix my social life." But "I'll send one text right now."

Why immediate? Because you're retraining your brain. Your brain just spent hours getting a fake reward (the fantasy). You need to give it a real reward (actual value-aligned action) as quickly as possible so it starts learning a new pattern.

Old pattern:
Feel discomfort → Drift into fantasy → Get simulated reward

New pattern:
Feel discomfort → Notice it → Anchor → Identify the value →
Take real action toward that value → Get real reward

You're not going to perfect this pattern overnight. But every time
you complete the cycle—even after a relapse—you're
strengthening it.

The 24-Hour Rule

Here's an important guideline for post-relapse recovery: **You
have 24 hours to get back on track.**

If you drift on Monday, that's a setback. If you drift Monday,
beat yourself up Tuesday, avoid your tools Wednesday, and give
up Thursday, that's a full relapse into the old pattern.

Don't let one bad day become a bad week.

Use the four-step plan within 24 hours of the drift:

1. Notice without drama
2. Anchor in your body
3. Get curious about the missing value
4. Take one small pivot action

Then get up the next day and return to your normal routine.
You're not starting over from scratch. You're just resuming the
path you were on. One detour doesn't mean you're lost.

Research on habit formation shows that missing one day doesn't
significantly impact long-term behavior change—but extended
lapses do (Lally et al., 2010). The difference between people
who ultimately succeed and people who give up often comes
down to how they handle the inevitable slip-ups. Do they spiral,
or do they recover quickly?

You're going to choose to recover quickly.

When to Adjust Your Plan

Sometimes a relapse is a sign that something in your plan needs adjusting.

If you're relapsing frequently:

- Are your anchoring techniques working? Maybe you need different ones.
- Are your Pivot actions too big? Maybe you need to make them smaller.
- Are you addressing the right values? Maybe you decoded your daydreams incorrectly.
- Are you under unusual stress? Maybe you need extra support right now.

This isn't about blame. It's about problem-solving. The tools in this book are flexible. If something isn't working, adjust it.

Maybe you need to check in with yourself more frequently (set more alarms).
Maybe you need more accountability (tell someone what you're working on).
Maybe you need to simplify your Pivot Plan (one action per week instead of three).
Maybe you need professional support (therapy can be helpful for some people).

Don't keep using a strategy that isn't working and then blame yourself when it doesn't work. That's insane. Change the strategy.

The Long View

Here's what you need to keep in mind: **recovery from MD isn't a straight line.**

You're not going to go from "constant daydreaming" to "perfect control" overnight. The actual trajectory looks something like this:

Weeks 1-2: High awareness, lots of relapses, but you're practicing the tools
Weeks 3-4: Catching yourself earlier, some successful redirects
Weeks 5-8: More good days than bad days, building confidence
Weeks 9-12: Occasional relapses, but quicker recovery
Months 4-6: Long stretches of control, with periodic setbacks
Months 6+: Daydreaming is manageable, life is more engaging

This is progress. It's messy, nonlinear, imperfect progress. But it's progress.

And every time you use the four-step relapse plan instead of spiraling into shame, you're reinforcing the new pattern. You're teaching your brain that setbacks aren't catastrophes. They're just information.

What You've Learned About Setbacks

Relapses are normal and predictable. They're part of the process, not proof that you're broken or that the approach doesn't work. What matters is how you respond when they happen.

The four-step relapse plan: Notice without drama, Anchor in your body, Get curious about the missing value, Make a new Pivot plan with one immediate small action. Complete this cycle within 24 hours of a relapse to prevent one bad day from becoming a bad week.

Self-compassion is more effective than self-criticism for sustained behavior change. Treat yourself like you'd treat a good friend who had a setback—with kindness and curiosity, not harsh judgment.

If you're relapsing frequently, adjust your plan. Make actions smaller, try different anchoring techniques, check if you're addressing the right values, or seek additional support. Don't keep using strategies that aren't working.

Recovery isn't linear. Expect messy, up-and-down progress over months. Every time you handle a setback well, you're building a stronger pattern and proving you can recover.

In the final chapter, we'll paint a picture of what life looks like when you're on the other side—not a life without daydreams, but a life where you're in control and your focus is anchored in a meaningful reality you've built.

Chapter 11: From Fantasy to Focus

Six months from now, maybe a year, maybe longer—the timeline doesn't matter—you're going to look up from your life and realize something has shifted.

You'll still daydream sometimes. Your imagination hasn't disappeared. But the compulsive pull is gone. The desperate need to escape has faded. You can choose when and how you engage with your fantasy world, and most of the time, you choose reality instead. Not because you're forcing yourself. Because reality is actually interesting now. There are things happening in your real life that you don't want to miss.

This is what recovery from maladaptive daydreaming looks like. Not perfection. Not a boring, imagination-free existence. Just **you, in charge of your own attention, living a life that doesn't require constant escape.**

Let's talk about what that life actually looks like and how you'll know you're getting there.

What "Recovered" Actually Means

First, let's clear up some misconceptions about recovery.

Recovery is NOT:

- Never daydreaming again
- Becoming someone who doesn't have a vivid imagination
- Having perfect focus and never getting distracted
- Solving all your problems and achieving your ideal life
- Feeling happy and fulfilled every single moment

Recovery IS:

- Being able to notice when you're drifting and redirect yourself most of the time
- Spending significantly less time in fantasy (hours per week instead of hours per day)
- Having a real life that feels meaningful enough that you don't desperately need escape
- Using your imagination intentionally for creative projects or problem-solving
- Feeling in control of your attention instead of controlled by your daydreams
- Handling stress and discomfort without automatically fleeing into fantasy
- Being present for the people and activities that matter to you

Recovery isn't about becoming a different person. It's about becoming a version of yourself who's grounded in reality while still having access to a rich inner life.

Research on addiction recovery—and MD operates on similar neural circuits—shows that successful recovery involves developing new coping strategies, rebuilding meaning and purpose in life, and creating a lifestyle that doesn't require the addictive behavior (Laudet, 2011). It's not about white-knuckling your way through cravings forever. It's about building a life where the cravings become less intense and less frequent because you're getting what you need from reality.

That's what we've been building throughout this book.

Signs You're Making Progress

How do you know it's working? What are the markers that you're moving in the right direction?

Early signs (Weeks 1-4):

- You're catching yourself drifting more quickly
- You're using the anchoring techniques at least sometimes
- You've identified your triggers and values
- You feel less shame about daydreaming because you understand it better
- You've taken at least a few values-based actions in real life

Middle signs (Months 2-4):

- Hours spent daydreaming per day have decreased noticeably
- You can resist some triggers that used to be automatic
- You're having more engaged conversations and present moments
- You're completing tasks that used to get derailed by drifting
- Your real life has some small areas of genuine satisfaction
- You're using scheduled creative time instead of just compulsive drifting

Later signs (Months 5+):

- You go multiple days without losing significant time to daydreaming
- When you do drift, you recover quickly using your tools
- You feel genuinely interested in real-life activities and relationships
- You have creative projects or hobbies that use your imagination productively
- People comment that you seem more present or engaged
- The fantasy world still exists but doesn't control you

The progression isn't perfectly linear. You'll have good weeks and bad weeks. But if you track your patterns over months, you should see the overall trajectory moving toward more control, more presence, more satisfaction with reality.

If you're not seeing any improvement after 2-3 months of consistent practice, that's a sign you need to adjust your approach or seek additional support (therapy, support groups, etc.).

What Real Life Feels Like Now

The most profound change isn't actually about the daydreaming. It's about how you experience your daily life.

Before, real life felt like:

- Something to get through until you could daydream again
- Boring, disappointing, not enough
- A constant reminder of what you're lacking
- Overwhelming and anxiety-inducing
- Lonely even when you were around people
- Like you were going through the motions without really living

Now, real life feels like:

- Something worth paying attention to
- Imperfect but genuine, with moments of real satisfaction
- A place where you're building things that matter
- Manageable, with tools to handle discomfort
- Connected, with some relationships where you're actually present
- Like you're participating, not just watching from the sidelines

You're not pretending everything is perfect. You're not delusionally optimistic. You're just... here. Present. Engaged with what's actually happening instead of constantly wishing you were somewhere else.

And that's the shift. You stop living in your head and start living in your life.

Your Imagination Has a New Job

Here's the best part: your vivid, creative imagination doesn't go to waste. It just has a new role.

You're still imaginative. You still have rich inner content. But now, instead of using your imagination to escape from your life, you're using it to *enhance* your life.

You might be:

- Writing stories or creating art based on your daydream content
- Using your imagination to problem-solve real challenges
- Engaging in structured creative activities (games, projects, hobbies)
- Planning future goals and visualizing how to achieve them
- Empathizing more deeply with others because you can imagine their perspectives
- Bringing creativity to your work or daily tasks

Your imagination is a tool you wield, not a force that wields you.

And here's something interesting: many people find that their creativity actually becomes *more* satisfying once they channel it into real projects. The fantasies were enjoyable but hollow— nothing came of them. But creating something tangible, something others can see or experience? That's genuinely fulfilling in a way fantasy never was.

Research on creativity and flow shows that people experience the deepest satisfaction when they're creating something real, with clear goals and immediate feedback (Csikszentmihalyi, 1990). Fantasy provides some pleasure, but it can't provide that sense of accomplishment that comes from finishing something, sharing it, getting responses.

Now you're getting that. And it feels better.

Relationships Are Different

One of the biggest changes you'll notice is in your relationships.

When you were deep in MD, you were only partly present with people. Half of you was there, nodding and making appropriate sounds. The other half was running through your mental storylines, waiting for the conversation to end so you could get back to the fantasy.

People probably sensed this, even if they couldn't name it. They might have said you seemed "distant" or "hard to reach."

Now, you're actually there. You're listening. You're responding authentically. You're present in the moment with them.

This changes everything.

Conversations become more satisfying because you're actually engaging. Friendships deepen because you're showing up. Family relationships improve because you're not constantly checked out. Romantic connections become possible because you're emotionally available.

You might even find that as you become more present, people are drawn to you more. Presence is attractive. Authenticity is magnetic. When you're genuinely *there*, people notice.

And the interesting thing is, real connection starts meeting that need that your romantic or social daydreams were trying to meet. You don't need to fantasize about being understood because you're experiencing actual understanding with real people. The fantasy loses its pull because reality is giving you the real thing.

Handling Stress Without Escape

One of the biggest tests of recovery is how you handle difficult times.

Before, any discomfort sent you straight into fantasy. Bad day at work? Daydream. Anxious about something? Daydream. Lonely weekend? Daydream.

Now, you have other tools. When stress hits, you:

- Notice the discomfort without immediately needing to escape it
- Anchor yourself physically to stay grounded
- Identify which value is being threatened
- Take a small action to address the real issue
- Or, if appropriate, sit with the discomfort without doing anything

This is huge. **You can be uncomfortable without fleeing.** That's emotional maturity. That's resilience.

You're not pretending life is easy. You're not toxic-positivity-ing your way through everything. You're just acknowledging, "This is hard right now, and I can handle it without checking out."

Sometimes you'll still want to escape. That urge doesn't completely disappear. But it's not the only option anymore. And most of the time, you choose to stay present and deal with reality instead.

Research on distress tolerance shows that people who can sit with uncomfortable emotions without avoiding them have better mental health outcomes across the board (Linehan, 2015). You're building that capacity. Every time you stay present through discomfort instead of fleeing into fantasy, you're proving to yourself that you can handle reality.

The Fantasy World Still Exists, But You're Not Living There

Your fantasy characters and storylines don't disappear. You might still think about them sometimes. You might still enjoy revisiting certain scenarios during your scheduled creative time.

The difference is, **you're visiting, not living there.**

You drop in, enjoy the mental movie for a bit, and then you leave. You don't move in for hours. You don't choose it over real activities and relationships. It's entertainment, inspiration, creative fuel—but it's not your primary residence anymore.

And honestly? It's probably more enjoyable now. When you're not desperately clinging to the fantasy as your only source of fulfillment, you can appreciate it for what it is—a fun mental playground, a creative resource, an interesting way your mind works.

Some people even find that their daydreams become less elaborate and less frequent naturally, without effort. When you're not feeding them constantly with your attention and emotional investment, they don't dominate your mental landscape the way they used to. They're just... there. Available if you want them. Not demanding if you don't.

133

You've Become Someone Who Follows Through

Here's something you might not expect: as you practice taking small values-based actions consistently, you start to see yourself differently.

You become someone who does what they say they'll do. Someone who finishes things. Someone who shows up.

This isn't just about the specific actions. It's about identity.

When you were lost in fantasy, you probably had lots of ideas and intentions but very little follow-through. You'd think about doing things, plan to do things, promise yourself you'd do things... and then drift into daydreaming instead. The gap between intention and action was huge.

Now, that gap has shrunk. You still imagine possibilities, but you also act on them. You start projects and complete them. You tell yourself you'll do something and then you actually do it.

This builds something psychologists call *self-efficacy*—the belief that you're capable of achieving what you set out to do (Bandura, 1997). And self-efficacy is one of the strongest predictors of success in any area of life. People who believe they're capable keep trying when things get hard. People who don't believe they're capable give up.

You're becoming someone who believes in their own capability. Not because you're perfect, but because you've proven to yourself through repeated small actions that you can follow through.

That's powerful.

The Life You've Built

So what does your life actually look like now, in concrete terms?

It varies for everyone, but here's what many people report:

At work or school:

- You're completing tasks in reasonable timeframes instead of avoiding them
- You're actually present in meetings and conversations
- You're proud of some of the work you've produced
- People see you as reliable and engaged

In relationships:

- You have a few genuine connections where you show up authentically
- You're not comparing real people to your fantasy ideals as much
- You can have meaningful conversations and actually remember them later
- People tell you they've noticed you seem more present

In your free time:

- You have real hobbies or creative pursuits you're actively engaged in
- You can enjoy activities without constantly wanting to be somewhere else
- You have some accomplishments or projects you're proud of
- You schedule creative time but aren't consumed by fantasy the rest of the day

In your inner life:

- You feel more grounded and in control of your attention

- You experience discomfort without immediately needing to escape
- You know your values and take actions aligned with them regularly
- You still have an active imagination but you're in charge of it

This isn't a perfect life. You still have problems, stress, disappointments. But it's a *real* life. One that you're actively building instead of perpetually escaping from.

And most days, that feels pretty good.

One Year from Now

Close your eyes for a moment and imagine: it's one year from today.

You wake up in the morning and instead of immediately drifting into fantasy, you get up. You go about your morning routine, present in your own life. Maybe you spend a few minutes writing, or sketching, or doing something creative you enjoy.

You go to work or school or whatever fills your day, and yeah, sometimes it's boring, sometimes it's hard. But you're there. You're handling it. You're not constantly checking out into mental movies. When you notice yourself starting to drift, you use your tools and come back.

You have lunch with a friend, or a coworker, or by yourself with a book. Either way, you're present. You're engaged with what's happening instead of with the storylines in your head.

The afternoon brings challenges—stress, tedium, frustration. You feel those emotions. You don't love them. But you don't immediately need to escape from them. You handle them. You take actions that matter. You stay.

In the evening, you have some creative time scheduled. You write for 30 minutes, or work on a project, or do something that uses your imagination productively. It feels good. Satisfying. You're creating something real.

Before bed, you reflect on the day. It wasn't perfect. There were hard moments. But you showed up. You were present. You moved toward what matters to you.

And you realize: this is enough. This real, imperfect, sometimes-difficult life is actually enough. You don't need to escape from it anymore.

That's where you're headed. Not to perfection. To presence. To a life that's worth showing up for.

The Journey You've Taken

Recovery from maladaptive daydreaming isn't about never daydreaming again. It's about being in control of your attention, spending far less time in fantasy, and building a real life that's meaningful enough that you don't desperately need escape.

You'll know you're making progress when you catch yourself drifting more quickly, use your tools consistently, spend fewer hours daydreaming, complete tasks you used to avoid, and start experiencing genuine satisfaction in real-life activities and relationships.

Real life starts to feel worth paying attention to—imperfect but genuine, with moments of real satisfaction. You stop living in your head and start living in your life. Your imagination has a new job: enhancing your life through creative projects, problem-solving, and bringing creativity to your daily existence.

Relationships improve dramatically as you become actually present with people. You can handle stress and discomfort without automatically fleeing into fantasy. You build self-efficacy by consistently following through on small actions, proving to yourself that you're capable.

The fantasy world still exists, but you're visiting, not living there. You've become someone who shows up, follows through, and builds a real life based on your values. Not a perfect life—a real life. And most days, that feels pretty good.

You have all the tools you need. The Anchor, the Pivot, the understanding of what drives you, the plan for when you stumble. Everything you need to reclaim your life from fantasy and build something real.

Now it's time to use them. Your life is waiting. And it's worth being present for.

References

- **Amabile, T. M., Hadley, C. N., & Kramer, S. J. (2002).** Creativity under the gun. *Harvard Business Review, 80*(8), 52–61.

- **Bandura, A. (1997).** *Self-efficacy: The exercise of control.* W. H. Freeman.

- **Bigelsen, J., Lehrfeld, J. M., Jopp, D. S., & Somer, E. (2016).** Maladaptive daydreaming: Evidence for an under-researched mental health issue. *Consciousness and Cognition, 42*, 254–266.

- **Bourne, E. J. (2015).** *The anxiety and phobia workbook* (6th ed.). New Harbinger Publications.

- **Brewer, J. A. (2017).** *The craving mind: From cigarettes to smartphones to love—Why we get hooked and how we can break bad habits.* Yale University Press.

- **Brewer, J. A., Worhunsky, P. D., Gray, J. R., Tang, Y.-Y., Weber, J., & Kober, H. (2011).** Meditation experience is associated with differences in default mode network activity and connectivity. *Proceedings of the National Academy of Sciences, 108*(50), 20254–20259.

- **Buckner, R. L., Andrews-Hanna, J. R., & Schacter, D. L. (2008).** The brain's default network: Anatomy, function, and relevance to disease. *Annals of the New York Academy of Sciences, 1124*(1), 1–38.

- **Burke, L. E., Wang, J., & Sevick, M. A. (2011).** Self-monitoring in weight loss: A systematic review of the literature. *Journal of the American Dietetic Association, 111*(1), 92–102.

- **Cooper, J. O., Heron, T. E., & Heward, W. L. (2020).** *Applied behavior analysis* (3rd ed.). Pearson.

- **Csikszentmihalyi, M. (1990).** *Flow: The psychology of optimal experience.* Harper & Row.

- **Doidge, N. (2007).** *The brain that changes itself: Stories of personal triumph from the frontiers of brain science.* Viking.

- **Gloster, A. T., Walder, N., Levin, M. E., Twohig, M. P., & Karekla, M. (2020).** The empirical status of acceptance and commitment therapy: A review of meta-analyses. *Journal of Contextual Behavioral Science, 18,* 181–192.

- **Gollwitzer, P. M., & Sheeran, P. (2006).** Implementation intentions and goal achievement: A meta-analysis of effects and processes. *Advances in Experimental Social Psychology, 38,* 69–119.

- **Griffiths, M. (2005).** A 'components' model of addiction within a biopsychosocial framework. *Journal of Substance Use, 10*(4), 191–197.

- **Harris, R. (2009).** *ACT made simple: An easy-to-read primer on acceptance and commitment therapy.* New Harbinger Publications.

- **Hayes, S. C., Strosahl, K. D., & Wilson, K. G. (2012).** *Acceptance and commitment therapy: The process and practice of mindful change* (2nd ed.). Guilford Press.

- **Killingsworth, M. A., & Gilbert, D. T. (2010).** A wandering mind is an unhappy mind. *Science, 330*(6006), 932.

- **Lally, P., van Jaarsveld, C. H. M., Potts, H. W. W., & Wardle, J. (2010).** How are habits formed: **Modelling** habit formation in the real world. *European Journal of Social Psychology, 40*(6), 998–1009.

- **Laudet, A. B. (2011).** The case for considering quality of life in addiction research and clinical practice. *Addiction Science & Clinical Practice, 6*(1), 44–55.

- **Lejuez, C. W., Hopko, D. R., Acierno, R., Daughters, S. B., & Pagoto, S. L. (2011).** Ten-year revision of the brief behavioral activation treatment for depression: Revised treatment manual. *Behavior Modification, 35*(2), 111–161.

- **Linehan, M. M. (2015).** *DBT skills training manual* (2nd ed.). Guilford Press.

- **Masuda, A., Hayes, S. C., Sackett, C. F., & Twohig, M. P. (2004).** Cognitive defusion and self-relevant negative thoughts: Examining the impact of a **ninety-year-old** technique. *Behaviour Research and Therapy, 42*(4), 477–485.

- **Najavits, L. M. (2001).** *Seeking Safety: A treatment manual for PTSD and substance abuse.* Guilford Press.

- **Neff, K. D., & Germer, C. K. (2013).** A pilot study and randomized controlled trial of the mindful self-compassion program. *Journal of Clinical Psychology, 69*(1), 28–44.

- **Ogden, P., Minton, K., & Pain, C. (2006).** *Trauma and the body: A sensorimotor approach to psychotherapy.* W. W. Norton & Company.

- **Porges, S. W. (2011).** *The polyvagal theory: Neurophysiological foundations of emotions, attachment, communication, and self-regulation.* W. W. Norton & Company.

- **Ryan, R. M., & Deci, E. L. (2000).** Self-determination theory and the facilitation of intrinsic motivation, social development, and well-being. *American Psychologist, 55*(1), 68–78.

- **Schultz, W. (2015).** Neuronal reward and decision signals: From theories to data. *Physiological Reviews, 95*(3), 853–951.

- **Schooler, J. W., Smallwood, J., Christoff, K., Handy, T. C., Reichle, E. D., & Sayette, M. A. (2011).** Meta-awareness, perceptual decoupling and the wandering mind. *Trends in Cognitive Sciences, 15*(7), 319–326.

- **Skinner, B. F. (1953).** *Science and human behavior.* Macmillan.

- **Smallwood, J., & Schooler, J. W. (2006).** The restless mind. *Psychological Bulletin, 132*(6), 946–958.

- **Somer, E. (2002).** Maladaptive daydreaming: A qualitative inquiry. *Journal of Contemporary Psychotherapy, 32*(2–3), 197–212.

- **Somer, E., Lehrfeld, J., Bigelsen, J., & Jopp, D. S. (2016).** Development and validation of the Maladaptive Daydreaming Scale (MDS). *Consciousness and Cognition, 39*, 77–91.

- **Somer, E., Soffer-Dudek, N., & Ross, C. A. (2017).** The comorbidity of daydreaming disorder (maladaptive daydreaming). *Journal of Nervous and Mental Disease, 205*(7), 525–530.

- **Tang, Y.-Y., Hölzel, B. K., & Posner, M. I. (2015).** The neuroscience of mindfulness meditation. *Nature Reviews Neuroscience, 16*(4), 213–225.

- **van der Kolk, B. A. (2014).** *The body keeps the score: Brain, mind, and body in the healing of trauma.* Viking.

- **Wegner, D. M., Schneider, D. J., Carter, S. R., & White, T. L. (1987).** Paradoxical effects of thought suppression. *Journal of Personality and Social Psychology, 53*(1), 5–13.

- **Wilson, K. G., & DuFrene, T. (2009).** *Mindfulness for two: An acceptance and commitment therapy approach to mindfulness in psychotherapy.* New Harbinger Publications.

www.ingramcontent.com/pod-product-compliance
Lightning Source LLC
Chambersburg PA
CBHW052012090426
42741CB00008B/1659